Mixed  'ch
for Nursing and
the Health Sciences

BRACKETT LIBRARY
6155 College Lane
Vero Beach, FL 32966

Mixed Methods Research for Nursing and the Health Sciences

Edited by

Sharon Andrew
PhD RN FRCNA
Head of Programme (Postgraduate Studies), School of Nursing
University of Western Sydney

and

Elizabeth J. Halcomb
RN BN(Hons) GradCert IntCareNurs PhD MRCNA
Senior Lecturer, School of Nursing
University of Western Sydney

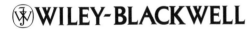

WILEY-BLACKWELL
A John Wiley & Sons, Ltd., Publication

This edition first published 2009
© 2009 by Blackwell Publishing Ltd

Blackwell Publishing was acquired by John Wiley & Sons in February 2007.
Blackwell's publishing programme has been merged with Wiley's global Scientific,
Technical, and Medical business to form Wiley-Blackwell.

Registered office
John Wiley & Sons Ltd, The Atrium, Southern Gate, Chichester, West Sussex,
PO19 8SQ, United Kingdom

Editorial offices
9600 Garsington Road, Oxford, OX4 2DQ, United Kingdom
2121 State Avenue, Ames, Iowa 50014-8300, USA

For details of our global editorial offices, for customer services and for information
about how to apply for permission to reuse the copyright material in this book please
see our website at www.wiley.com/wiley-blackwell.

The right of the authors to be identified as the authors of this work has been asserted
in accordance with the Copyright, Designs and Patents Act 1988.

All rights reserved. No part of this publication may be reproduced, stored in a
retrieval system, or transmitted, in any form or by any means, electronic, mechanical,
photocopying, recording or otherwise, except as permitted by the UK Copyright,
Designs and Patents Act 1988, without the prior permission of the publisher.

Wiley also publishes its books in a variety of electronic formats. Some content that
appears in print may not be available in electronic books.

Designations used by companies to distinguish their products are often claimed as
trademarks. All brand names and product names used in this book are trade names,
service marks, trademarks or registered trademarks of their respective owners.
The publisher is not associated with any product or vendor mentioned in this book.
This publication is designed to provide accurate and authoritative information in
regard to the subject matter covered. It is sold on the understanding that the publisher
is not engaged in rendering professional services. If professional advice or other expert
assistance is required, the services of a competent professional should be sought.

Library of Congress Cataloging-in-Publication Data

Mixed methods research for nursing and the health sciences / edited by Sharon Andrew, Elizabeth Halcomb.
p. ; cm.
Includes bibliographical references and index.
ISBN 978-1-4051-6777-2 (pbk. : alk. paper)   1. Nursing–Research–Methodology.
2. Medical sciences–Research–Methodology.   3. Qualitative research.
4. Quantitative research.   I. Halcomb, Elizabeth.   II. Title.
[DNLM: 1. Nursing Research–methods.   2. Data Collection.   3. Health Services
Research–methods.   4. Research Design. WY 20.5 A563m 2009]
RT81.5.A53 2009
610.73072–dc22
2008028170

A catalogue record for this book is available from the British Library.

Set in 10 on 12 pt Palatino by SNP Best-set Typesetter Ltd., Hong Kong
Printed and bound in Malaysia by KHL Printing Co Sdn Bhd

1   2009

3 2903 30059 9799

Table of Contents

Foreword

Contemporary health care systems face a myriad of problems requiring collaboration among health professions and the use of a range of methodological and epistemological approaches. Often solving these complex dilemmas also requires a partnership between social, health and human scientists. Fortunately, these challenges in contemporary society have also increased the receptivity of funding bodies to study designs that use interdisciplinary approaches and develop innovative, yet rigorous, approaches to scholarly enquiry. An exciting development within this current milieu is that nursing and health services research has truly come of age and frequently nurse scientists partner with a range of professionals to work on solutions to improve the health and well-being of individuals, their families and the broader society.

Mixed methods research is a systematic approach to addressing research questions that involve collecting, analysing and synthesising both quantitative and qualitative data in a single research project. The success of the mixed methods approach in addressing complex study questions has led to increasing interest and adaptation of these methods. In parallel to the increased usage has also been the increasing refinement of methodological and pragmatic issues.

The editors of, and contributors to, *Mixed Methods Research for Nursing and the Health Sciences* provide the reader with an accessible, scholarly and pragmatic guide for undertaking mixed methods research. This text targeting the novice and postgraduate researcher is a valuable addition to the scholarly debate and discussion of mixed methods research.

The novice researcher is often perplexed and frustrated by a range of terminology. This text not only provides clear definitions of terminology used in mixed methods research but also provides the reader with pragmatic tips in managing the research process. In Chapter 2, Muncey provides the reader with a foundation understanding of the theoretical and philosophical underpinnings of mixed methods research, while in Chapter 5 Brannen and Halcomb explore sampling and data collection methods. Subsequent chapters provide insight into methodological rigour in data collection and analysis. Bazeley, in Chapter 6, provides information on innovative ways to integrate datasets in mixed methods designs while, in Chapter 7, Giddings and Grant demonstrate how the concepts of validity, reliability and rigour are applied in mixed methods designs.

Part Three of *Mixed Methods Research for Nursing and the Health Sciences* provides an exciting contribution to the discussion of mixed methods and examples of applying theoretical and conceptual issues of mixed methods research in practice. In Chapter 9, Creswell et al. illustrate important considerations in applying mixed methods in intervention trials. The pragmatic examples in this section should inspire researchers, both experienced and novice, to explore mixed methods principles in their own research.

The editors, Andrew and Halcomb, are to be congratulated on their collaborative approach in engaging a range of experienced and novice mixed methods researchers in writing this informative and engaging text. This range of perspectives increases the applicability and relevance of this important textbook.

I enthusiastically commend this text for both experienced and novice researchers as well as health professionals engage in clinical practice. *Mixed Methods Research for Nursing and the Health Sciences* will, I am sure, inspire and motivate a range of novel approaches to addressing important issues facing health care providers and consumers.

Patricia M. Davidson RN PhD
Professor of Cardiovascular and Chronic Care
Curtin University of Technology
Sydney, Australia

Preface

Purpose of this book

Striving to bridge the chasm between the quantitative and qualitative paradigms, mixed methods research has developed to become a rational and conceptually congruent method to explain phenomena that are complex and multifaceted. Research problems faced by researchers in the modern world often require qualitative and quantitative methods to not only explore and describe but also assess and evaluate. The science of mixed methods research has forged this new path that combines both methods within a single study observing theoretical and methodological congruence. Researchers from nursing and the health sciences, in particular, have sought to embrace mixed methods to help explain the complex phenomena that influence human health. Just as there is a need to consider the theoretical underpinnings and careful planning of data collection methods and analysis techniques in the discrete approaches of quantitative and qualitative research, similarly mixed methods research needs to be well designed to provide rigorous data.

Despite the growth in popularity of mixed methods investigations in nursing and health sciences research, there is a dearth of debate that focuses specifically on the unique issues faced by researchers working with this research design, particularly focusing on pragmatic issues. Therefore, this book aims to provide much needed scholarly and practical discourse related to the design, conduct and reporting of mixed methods research in nursing and the health sciences.

Intended audience

This book targets the postgraduate research student/beginning researcher (clinician) level. However, it will also serve as a useful reference source for undergraduate research students who are seeking to develop an understanding of mixed methods research. Additionally, academics will be able to use the text as a reference resource for conducting and teaching mixed methods research. This text provides practical advice for researchers to assist them in navigating the various phases of planning, conducting and reporting mixed methods research, including how to ensure that the project maintains sufficient rigour for external review. Through this information we seek to provide answers to questions or issues that continually arise from our research students, during workshops and at conferences. The use of international published studies as examples and engagement of contributors from across the globe will help to assure the applicability of the text to a wide audience.

We have attempted to provide a practical guide to implementing mixed methods research specifically in health services research. We have intentionally resisted pressure to confine the content to a specific health discipline. This was felt to be especially important given that the issues raised in the text have a broad application for researchers, both within health (e.g. nursing, medical, allied health) and related disciplines (e.g. social sciences), particularly given the increase in interdisciplinary collaborative research being undertaken within the health care sector. Further we have avoided the temptation to focus solely on theoretical elements, rather using the opportunity to provide tangible, real world examples.

Features of the book

The content of the book has been arranged to facilitate use by the researcher in planning a mixed methods investigation or by students and academics in the course of a workshop or research methods programme. The framework behind the book is that of a generic research process including understanding the methodological and conceptual approach, designing the study, conducting the investigation, reporting the results, and maintaining auditable, ethical and accountable research practice. Although this is clearly an oversimplification of the process, it follows the well recognised research process making it accessible to the reader and a template for future investigations.

Throughout the book, contributors have designed hints (points of reflection) and provided summaries of key points and key terms. This approach has reinforced the main points of each of the chapters and is intended to stimulate and provoke critical reflection. Where possible, research examples from the peer-reviewed literature have also been cited to illustrate key points from the chapter and provide practical examples. Additionally, contributors have generously provided important insights into their own experiences of using mixed methods principles in their own research programmes, providing both novice and expert researchers with useful information.

Book contributors

We are very privileged to have assembled such an accomplished group of health care researchers from a range of backgrounds with expertise in mixed methods research. The contributors are a truly international group, with representation from Australia, New Zealand, the United Kingdom and the United States and across a range of disciplines. All contributors have significant experience in conducting mixed methods research within their own research programmes and have published related papers in the peer-reviewed literature. The diversity of perspectives that such a group has brought to the text has been refreshing and enlightening.

Acknowledgements

The completion of this book would not have been possible without the dedicated and enthusiastic work of our contributors. We sincerely appreciate the contribution that each has made to the development of this book and to our further understanding of mixed methods research.

Our work on this book has benefited significantly from the contributions of many of our colleagues. Special thanks to Professor Patricia Davidson, Curtin University of Technology, for her foreword for this book and her critical appraisal of our chapters. As members of the University of Western Sydney School of Nursing N-FORCE research group we offer special thanks for the practical and collegial support of Professor Debra Jackson and the members of N-FORCE who have pioneered many of the applications of mixed methods research. Also to Yenna Salamonson for her encouragement to write this text.

This innovative and practical text is poised at an exciting time in the evolution of mixed methods research. We anticipate this being a useful text for researchers planning and conducting mixed methods studies in nursing and the health sciences.

Sharon Andrew & Elizabeth J. Halcomb

Editors and Contributors

Editors

Sharon Andrew RN RM DipAppSc(NursEd) BAppSc MSc(Hons) PhD
  FRCNA
Senior Lecturer and Head of Programme (Postgraduate Studies), School
  of Nursing, University of Western Sydney, New South Wales,
  AUSTRALIA

Elizabeth J. Halcomb RN BN(Hons) Grad Cert IC PhD MRCNA
Senior Lecturer School of Nursing, University of Western Sydney, New
  South Wales, AUSTRALIA

Contributors

Patricia Bazeley BA(Hons) PhD
Director and consultant, Research Support P/L, Bowral NSW,
  AUSTRALIA
Senior Research Fellow, Quality of Life and Social Justice Research
  Centre, Australian Catholic University, Fitzroy, Vic., AUSTRALIA

Julia Brannen MSc PhD FRSA AcSS
Professor in the Sociology of the Family, Thomas Coram Research Unit,
  Institute of Education, University of London, Adjunct Professor at

the University of Bergen, Norway, and Co-Founder and Co-Editor of *The International Journal of Social Research Methodology*, UNITED KINGDOM

John Creswell PhD
Professor of Educational Psychology, Co-Director, Office of Qualitative and Mixed Methods Research, and Founding Co-Editor, *Journal of Mixed Methods Research*, University of Nebraska-Lincoln, Lincoln, Nebraska, UNITED STATES OF AMERICA

Patricia M. Davidson RN PhD
Professor, School of Nursing and Midwifery, Curtin University of Technology, Sydney Campus, AUSTRALIA

Michael D. Fetters MD MPH MA
Associate Professor, Department of Family Medicine, Director, Japanese Family Health Program, University of Michigan, UNITED STATES OF AMERICA

Lynne S. Giddings RGON MN PhD
Associate Professor, School of Nursing, Faculty of Health & Environmental Sciences, AUT University, Auckland, Aotearoa, NEW ZEALAND

Donna Gillies PhD
Research Officer, Mental Health Nursing Research Unit, University of Western Sydney and Sydney West Area Health Service, AUSTRALIA

Barbara M. Grant PhD
Centre for Academic Development, The University of Auckland, Auckland, Aotearoa, NEW ZEALAND

Thilo Kroll PhD
Senior Lecturer, Alliance for Self Care Research, School of Nursing & Midwifery, University of Dundee, Scotland, UNITED KINGDOM

Reshin Maharaj RN PhD (candidate)
School of Nursing, University of Western Sydney
Clinical Nurse Specialist, Cumberland Hospital, AUSTRALIA

Alejandro Morales MA PhD (candidate)
Department of Educational Psychology, University of Nebraska-Lincoln, Lincoln, Nebraska, UNITED STATES OF AMERICA

Tessa Muncey RN RHV NDN Cert Cert Ed BA(Hons) MA PhD
Senior Lecturer, University of Leeds, UNITED KINGDOM

Melinda T. Neri BA
Research Analyst, School of Nursing, Department of Social and Behavioural Sciences, University of California, San Francisco (UCSF), UNITED STATES OF AMERICA

Louise O'Brien RN PhD
Associate Professor of Nursing, Mental Health Nursing Research Unit, University of Western Sydney and Sydney West Area Health Service, AUSTRALIA

Alicia O'Cathain PhD
Senior Research Fellow, School of Health and Related Research (ScHARR), University of Sheffield, Sheffield, UNITED KINGDOM

Jane Phillips RN PhD
Programme Manager, Quality and Professional Development Cancer Australia, Lyneham ACT, AUSTRALIA

Vicki L. Plano Clark PhD
Research Assistant, Professor of Educational Psychology, Co-Director, Office of Qualitative and Mixed Methods Research, and Managing Editor, *Journal of Mixed Methods Research*, University of Nebraska-Lincoln, Lincoln, Nebraska, UNITED STATES OF AMERICA

Glossary

Action research – A research design that encompasses critical reflection and action, where the participants and researcher work together to implement change.

After-trial mixed methods intervention study – The collection of qualitative data after the intervention has been concluded. This qualitative data can be used to help explain within- and between-subject variations in outcomes, verify individual scores on outcomes measures and note discrepancies between the planned intervention and its actual approach.

Before-trial mixed methods intervention study – The collection of qualitative data before an intervention that is used to support the intervention, such as helping to select participants for the trial or helping to develop the intervention.

Catalytic validity – Refers to the extent to which the research contributes to social change.

Concurrent mixed methods design – A design in which the qualitative and quantitative data are collected at the same time, but independently of each other. The final study results are based on the findings from both sets of data.

Concurrent nested design – In this study design, one of the data collection methods dominates and the other one is embedded in it with all data collected at the same time.

Concurrent transformative design – A design in which the qualitative and quantitative data collection are informed by specified theory, with all the data collected at the same time.

Concurrent triangulated design – This design involves a single study containing qualitative and quantitative data collection which are conducted at the same time and each method seeks to validate the evidence produced by the other.

Data transformation – Involves the conversion of data from one form to another.

Design – The overall approach to a study which encompasses the aim, methods and the anticipated outcomes (Thurston 2006).

Design validity – In experimental research the study needs to be designed in such a way as to reduce the threats to internal validity and external validity.

During-trial mixed methods intervention study – The collection of qualitative data while an intervention is in progress that provides qualitative information for comparison to the quantitative data. In some studies, the qualitative data focus on the experiences of the participants during the intervention while the quantitative data provide information about the outcomes.

Evidence-based practice – Practice which is based upon a combination of the best available research evidence, clinician experience and consumer/community preferences.

Generalisability – The degree to which we can infer the findings from the research sample to the population.

Integrated model – Reporting all methods in one chapter and having results chapters based on themes which each draw on data from either the qualitative or quantitative component or both of these.

Integration – The 'knitting together' of different approaches to research within any or all of the components of a study.

Measurement validity – Refers to the way that the tools or instruments are constructed and how they are used.

Meta-analysis – Statistical or other strategy applied to the analysis of multiple data from several sources of data or several studies.

Metamatrix – Tabulation of summary data derived from different sources and often of different types, to facilitate analysis of patterns across those different sources.

Method – The steps taken by the researcher(s) to collect the data for a specific study. These are the 'doing tools', that is, the way data are collected and analysed (Giddings and Grant 2007). For example: survey, interview or focus group.

Methodology – The approach used by the researcher(s) to guide the conduct of the study. The methodology is the 'thinking tool', the worldview (paradigm) that influences how a researcher presents a research question, and decides on the methods and data analysis to employ in a study (Giddings and Grant 2007). For example: phenomenology, grounded theory or randomised control trial.

Mixed methods – The use of both qualitative and quantitative methods of data collection in a single study. For example, combining qualitative interviews and quantitative survey data collection.

Mixed methods analysis – Strategies in which the researcher describes, compares and relates ideas embedded in multiple data sources or derived through multiple analytical strategies, and interprets these in the light of the data as a whole.

Mixed methods research – This form of enquiry is seen as both a methodology and a method. As a methodology it has philosophical assumptions – often based in pragmatism – that guide the direction of the collection, analysis and mix of research in all phases of the enquiry. As a method, it involves collecting, analysing and mixing both quantitative and qualitative data in a single study or a series of studies.

Multi-method research – The use of two or more data collection methods from the same research tradition. For example, participant observation and interviews (qualitative), or survey and population census data (quantitative).

Paradigm – The philosophical underpinnings from which specific research approaches stem (e.g. positivism, pragmatism).

Positivism – This structured methodological perspective views research as an objective, empirical process that is independent of the researcher's influences.

Pragmatism – A philosophical stance that embraces multiple viewpoints of a research problem. It is the proposed methodological basis for mixed methods research.

Priority – The level of importance given to each type of data collection.

Qualitised data – Numerical data converted into narrative format.

Quantitised data – Qualitative coding converted into numerical form, for statistical analysis.

Randomised controlled trial – An experimental study in which participants are randomly allocated to either the intervention or control group.

Reliability – The degree of consistency with which a research tool measures what it is supposed to measure.

Research design – A planned systematic approach that incorporates the aims, methods and expected outcomes for a research project.

Rigour – The thoroughness, accuracy, confirmability and ethical soundness of all aspects of a study's design.

Segregated models – Reporting components of a study separately, using one chapter to report the qualitative component and another chapter to report the quantitative component.

Self-reflexivity – Involves processes of ensuring the integrity and credibility of the interpretive researcher.

Sequential mixed methods design – A design where the findings from one type of data collection method (e.g. survey) is followed by another type of data collection method (e.g. interviews), with the findings based on an integration of both datasets.

Sequential explanatory design – A design typically comprises a quantitative data collection phase followed by a qualitative phase that seeks to assist in explaining the quantitative findings.

Sequential exploratory design – This design is undertaken when little is known about a phenomenon and typically begins with a qualitative phase followed by a quantitative phase.

Sequential transformative design – A design in which the qualitative and quantitative data collection is informed by specified theory, with one type of data collection (e.g. interviews) subsequently followed by another type of data collection (e.g. surveys).

Synthesis – Placing diverse sources of data under a common framework to facilitate pattern analysis.

Triangulation – The use of two or more data sources, investigators, methods or theories in the study of a phenomenon. This may or may not involve the combination of qualitative and quantitative methods of data collection in a single study.

Trustworthiness – The degree of confidence that the researcher has that their qualitative data and findings are credible, transferable and dependable.

Validation – An umbrella concept for processes which ensure quality, or rigour, in research.

Validity – The degree to which a research tool measures what it is supposed to measure.

The editors would like to acknowledge that the terms in this glossary have been compiled from material supplied by a number of the book's contributors.

References

Giddings L.S. and Grant B.M. (2007) A Trojan horse for positivism? A critique of mixed methods. *Advances in Nursing Science*, **30**, 52–60.

Thurston W., Cove L. and Meadows L.M. (2006) Methodological congruence in complex and collaborative mixed method projects. *International Journal of Multiple Research Approaches*, 2(1), 2–14.

Section One
Preliminary Considerations

Introduction to Mixed Methods Research for Nursing and the Health Sciences

Elizabeth J. Halcomb, Sharon Andrew and Julia Brannen

> ### Learning objectives
>
> After reading this chapter, you will have an understanding of the:
>
> a) Research process related to mixed methods research in nursing and the health sciences.
> b) Current trends in nursing and health sciences research, including the changes in the nature of research (for example: the complexities of research problems, requirements of funding bodies) and support for new approaches to research.
> c) Key terms used in mixed methods research including a definition of mixed methods.

Introduction

In recent years there has been an increased interest in formal mixed methods research, although for many years researchers have reported the findings of qualitative and qualitative data collection methods within the one study. As a methodology, mixed methods is more than simply the ad hoc combination of qualitative and quantitative data in a single study. It involves the planned mixing of qualitative and quantitative methods at a predetermined stage of the research process, be it during the initial study planning, the process of data collection, data analysis or reporting, in order to better answer the research question.

Mixed methods research has reached a critical point in its evolution. A growing body of literature debates the philosophy behind using mixed methods and reports the findings of studies conducted using mixed methods designs. However, this body of literature seldom provides detailed descriptions of the practical aspects of how the mixing of methods can be rigorously achieved. Additionally, our observations, from a range of conferences and meetings where mixed methods research has been presented, identify significant issues in the implementation of mixed methods designs, particularly concerning the ways of integrating mixed methods data and the presentation of study findings. To ensure that mixed methods research is considered as rigorous as qualitative or quantitative designs, it is essential that those implementing it consider the implications of their methodological choices. This is not to say that there is only one way of conducting mixed methods research; indeed, researcher creativity is an important component of mixed methods designs. However, adequate planning must be undertaken to ensure rigour and quality within the project.

This book aims to provide a practical guide to conducting mixed methods research in nursing and the health sciences, and importantly outlines processes for methodological rigour. As such, it will provide much needed scholarly and practical discourse related to the design, conduct and reporting of mixed methods research in nursing and health sciences research.

Organisation of the book

Mixed methods is a relatively new design for many researchers, and it is necessary to introduce the approach, provide specific guidance relating to how to implement the design and information about the specific procedures involved (Creswell and Plano Clark 2006). This book seeks to provide this information to the researcher in a practical format, relating the philosophical and methodological considerations of mixed methods research with practical advice as to how these considerations can be implemented in nursing and health sciences research. Figure 1.1 depicts the three sections and twelve chapters of the text. Section One consists of four chapters that discuss the preliminary considerations in using mixed methods research in contemporary nursing and health sciences research. Section Two contains four chapters, each of which describes a specific aspect of the research process in a mixed methods investigation. Section Three consists of the final three chapters that describe how mixed methods has been implemented in intervention trials, action research and a sequential triangulated mixed methods design, and contains the concluding chapter which highlights contemporary and future issues for mixed methods researchers.

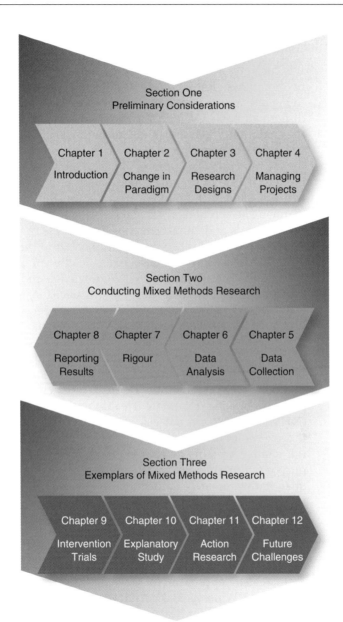

Figure 1.1 Structure of the text. (Figure designed by J. Rolley.)

Current trends in nursing and health sciences research

It is currently an exciting time in health service delivery across a range of disciplines. Rapid social change, the pressures of contemporary living, an ageing population and an increase in complex and chronic disease all have a significant impact on the health and well-being of the community (Andrew and Halcomb 2006). Such issues also impact upon the delivery of health care and have created an urgent need to review the roles of various clinician groups, service delivery and models of care to promote the delivery of best practice interventions that will deliver the optimal treatment in the most resource efficient manner. The spiralling costs of the health care system are forcing health professionals to demonstrate the effectiveness of their interventions in terms of the cost to the system and benefit to the patient (Gaziano et al. 2007). To accomplish these goals, health care professionals need to access and critically analyse new knowledge and, where appropriate, incorporate the findings into clinical decision making (Wirtz et al. 2006). Mixed methods research offers a way of conducting research that will meet the needs of health care professionals.

Contemporary health care is increasingly seeking to implement evidence-based practice across disciplines. Although evidence can be drawn from a diverse range of sources, it is generally accepted that the findings of methodologically rigorous research are optimal for guiding decision making (National Health and Medical Research Council (NHMRC) 2007). Once it is accepted that research evidence is required to seek a solution to a clinical dilemma, then the debate centres around the relative weights of each methodological approach. It is not the purpose of this chapter to debate the relative merits of qualitative and quantitative research. Rather, this chapter seeks to assert, that for some research problems a mixed methods approach is the optimal means of providing a balanced approach to understanding the relative issues and their impact on the research problem. The multifaceted nature of the phenomena that contemporary health care professionals are concerned with investigating frequently demands the use of a similarly multifaceted approach to develop understandings and insights (Coyle and Williams 2000; Andrew and Halcomb 2006) and increase the evidence base for health care practitioners (Flemming 2007). Mixed methods research offers a means by which to achieve this aim whilst still providing a rigorous methodological framework (Andrew and Halcomb 2006).

When considering the role of mixed methods research it is also important to consider the transcendence of paradigms. Some health care researchers are concerned with generating understandings at the micro level while others are concerned with the macro level. Those in the former group emphasise the agency of those they study through an emphasis upon studying the subjective interpretations and perspectives of individuals. However those working at the macro level are concerned with larger-scale patterns and trends and seek to pose structural explanations. Despite this observation all health care researchers aim to understand groups or individuals in society. If one is to conceptually transcend the micro and the macro levels, then methods must be developed to reflect this transcendence (Kelle 2001). Thus the application of qualitative and quantitative methods may depend upon the extent to which researchers seek to produce different levels and types of explanation. Whether these levels of explanation are commensurable may become less important than the fact of bringing them together.

Impetus towards a greater use of mixed methods

Despite evidence that the *'paradigm wars'* between qualitative and quantitative research are still in progress, the use of a combination of methods, whether within a single paradigm (multimethod) or across paradigms (mixed methods), is becoming an increasingly accepted research approach (Bryman 2006). At the same time it is important to recognise that the underpinning of mixed methods research is nothing new but has always been part, at least implicitly, of many researchers' repertoires particularly in the health sciences. What are new, are the emerging impetuses that are leading researchers to methodological change and advancement. Where previously people were reluctant to disclose this combination of approaches, researchers are now discussing frank and meaningful information regarding methodological issues leading to innovation and the greater potential to have a repertoire of skills appropriate to a range of research questions.

The impetus driving healthcare researchers to critically analyse their methods comes from many directions, including: 1) increased reflexivity about researcher–researched relationships; 2) increased political awareness about what and who research is for; 3) growing formalisation of research governance and ethics procedures; 4) the availability and ease of new technologies; and 5) international research collaboration (Brannen 1992; Brannen 2008). Such forces are likely to make researchers reconsider their tried and tested ways of doing research and to invest in a range of innovative data collection methods.

Increased reflexivity in relationships

The increased evidence of sensitivity and reflexivity on the part of nursing and health science researchers may reshape their choices about research methods. As some argue, reflexivity is not solely about checking for researcher effects but also refers to researchers' relationships with those whom they seek to study, and how researchers themselves relate to both the research methods and to other members of the research team (Koch and Harrington 1998; Northway 2000). Giddings and Grant (2007) caution that mixed methods researchers must use and report their reflexivity in their research, as omission of this information may lead to the suspicion of mixed methods research as a 'trojan horse for positivism'.

Increased political awareness

A second impetus concerns the increased emphasis on the politics of research and the research process. At one end of the spectrum, there is a demand that all research, at least to some degree, be useful in terms of policy making and/or clinical practice development. In Chapter 2, Muncey elaborates how 'useful' has tended to be synonymous with the quantitative paradigm where randomised controlled trials are accepted as the gold standard. Moreover, this type of research is favoured by major funding organisations. Further along the spectrum are 'participatory methods' where the emphasis is on social awareness and change by giving a voice to the gendered, disadvantaged and disempowered groups. In recent years, participatory methods have become increasingly popular in nursing research.

Growing formalisation of research governance

A third impetus to methodological change concerns research governance and ethics. Choice of research methods has always been open to ethical scrutiny in terms of their effects on research participants. However, formal frameworks for research governance are increasingly being implemented, with an expansion in mandatory Human Research Ethics Committees through which researchers have to seek permission to conduct their research. In addition to institutional human research ethics committees, researchers may also need to meet the requirements of funding bodies and the agencies that provide access to potential participants. Such processes may significantly influence the researchers' choice of research method. This may prompt the researcher to adopt mixed methods research designs when they previously would have conducted a purely qualitative or quantitative investigation. In Chapter 9, Creswell and colleagues discuss how a randomised controlled trial can incorporate qualitative data to develop a mixed approach to a study.

New technologies

A fourth impetus that may more directly influence the range of methods employed in researchers' repertoires has to do with the potential for methodological innovation created following the development, expansion and refinement of new technology. The integration of data so that it is truly 'mixed', to form a hybrid of numbers and words, is a real possibility with computer programs such as NVivo. In Chapter 6, Bazeley discusses the role of computer technology to integrate and analyse mixed methods data. Other technologies are discussed by Brannen and Halcomb in Chapter 5.

International research collaboration

There is growing interest in international research collaboration, which has occurred as globalisation and international issues attract greater attention. Additionally, funding bodies are increasingly calling for international partnerships for specific projects. Cross-national research often requires a number of different data sources. Such data sources are likely to emanate from a range of very different methods of data collection and need to be considered within the parameters of cultural acceptability and appropriateness.

Mixed methods terminology

What is mixed methods research?

Although the notion of mixing data has been in existence for around 40 years there have been significant developments not only in the science but also in the terminology of mixed methods research. From its early nomenclature of multiple operationalism (Campbell and Fiske 1959) to triangulation (Jick 1979), between-method triangulation (Denzin 1989) and multimethod research (Brewer and Hunter 1989), the term mixed methods has emerged. In this book we have adopted the simple definition of mixed methods as research which collects both qualitative and quantitative data in the one study and integrates these data at some stage of the research process. This definition is expanded and developed in the chapters of the book. For example, in Chapter 2 Muncey defines and debates the paradigm issues related to mixed methods. In the final chapter, Andrew and Halcomb present their views on how this definition can be refined to incorporate the debates and contemporary developments in mixed methods research.

We have adopted Tashakkori and Teddlie's (2003) definition of 'multimethod' research as being a combination of methods from the same paradigm. The distinction between mixed methods and multi-method research is illustrated in Box 1.1.

Box 1.1 Research in action

A mixed methods study of caregiver grief used (qualitative) interviews informed by descriptive phenomenology and (quantitative) standardised instruments to measure distress and grief while caring for a person with a terminal illness and during bereavement (Waldrop 2007).

A multimethod study used observation and interviews to explore maternal experiences of using kangaroo holding in a neonatal intensive care unit (Johnson 2007).

Methods versus methodology

Methods and methodology are other terms that are frequently used (or abused) by researchers. In this text we prefer the definitions proposed by Giddings and Grant (2007) where methodology is defined as a 'thinking tool' that is the worldview (paradigm) that influences how a researcher presents a research question, and decides on the methods and data analysis to employ in a study. Methods, by comparison, are considered the 'doing tools', i.e. the way data are collected and analysed (Giddings and Grant 2007). For example, a phenomenological study used interviews to explore the lived experience of the ICU nurse caring for clients having treatment withdrawn or withheld (Halcomb et al. 2004). The methodology would be phenomenology, whilst the method would be semi-structured interviews.

Research design

Another term used throughout the book is research design. The design is the overall approach to a study which encompasses the aim, methods and the anticipated outcomes (Thurston 2006). A research design should be congruent with the methodology chosen for the study. Research designs in mixed methods are varied and Kroll and Neri present some popular mixed methods designs and practical considerations for their implementation in Chapter 3. In Chapters 9, 10 and 11 examples of research designs are presented. Creswell and colleagues present a mixed methods design that combines qualitative data with a randomised controlled trial in Chapter 9. The latter two chapters are based on doctoral programmes where the primary authors have adopted a multistage mixed methods approach. These chapters have been included, not only as exemplars, but also to provide encouragement to other higher degree students and researchers who have taken the mixed methods path. We hope this book will assist you with some of those practical decisions on your research journey.

Conclusion

In this chapter we have introduced the reader to the current trends in mixed methods research, and to the terminology that will be expanded and refined during progress through the text. We wish you well in your research and studies and look forward to watching the science of mixed methods develop and grow in the future.

References

Andrew S. and Halcomb E.J. (2006) Mixed methods research is an effective method of enquiry for working with families and communities. *Contemporary Nurse*, **23**, 145–153.

Brannen J. (1992) *Mixing Methods: Qualitative and Quantitive Research*. Aldershot: Bower.

Brannen J. (2008) The practice of a mixed methods research strategy: personal, professional and project considerations in Bergman M. (ed.) *Advances in Mixed Methods Research: Theories and applications*. London: Sage Publications.

Brewer J. and Hunter A. (1989) *Multimethod Research: A Synthesis of Styles*. New York: Sage Publications.

Bryman A. (2006) Paradigm peace and the implication for quality. *International Journal of Social Research Methodology*, **9**, 111–126.

Campbell D.T. and Fiske D.W. (1959) Convergent and discriminant validation by the multitrait–multimethod matrix. *Psychological Bulletin*, **56**, 81–105.

Coyle J. and Williams B. (2000) An exploration of the epistemological intricacies of using qualitative data to develop a quantitative measure of user views of health care. *Journal of Advanced Nursing*, **31**, 1235–1243.

Creswell J.W. and Plano Clark V. (2006) *Designing and Conducting Mixed Methods Research.* Thousand Oaks, California: Sage Publications.

Denzin N. (1989) *The Research Art: A Theoretical Introduction of Sociological Methods*, 3rd edition. Chicago: Aldine.

Flemming K. (2007) The knowledge base for evidence-based nursing: a role for mixed methods research. *Advances in Nursing Science*, **30**, 41–51.

Gaziano T.A., Galea G. and Reddy K.S. (2007) Scaling up interventions for chronic disease prevention: the evidence. *Lancet*, **370**, 1939–1946.

Giddings L.S. and Grant B.M. (2007) A trojan horse for positivism? A critique of mixed methods. *Advances in Nursing Science*, **30**, 52–60.

Halcomb E.J., Daly J., Jackson D. and Davidson P. (2004) An insight into Australian nurses' experience of withdrawal/withholding of treatment in the ICU. *Intensive and Critical Care Nursing*, **20**, 214–222.

Jick T.D. (1979) Mixing qualitative and quantitative methods: triangulation in action. *Administrative Science Quarterly*, **24**, 602–611.

Johnson A.N. (2007) The maternal experience of kangaroo holding. *JOGNN: Journal of Obstetric, Gynecologic, and Neonatal Nursing*, **36**, 568–573.

Kelle U. (2001) Sociological explanations between micro and macro and the integration of qualitative and quantitative methods. *Forum: Qualitative Social Research*, **2**, http://www.qualitative-research.net/fqs-texte/1-01/1-01kelle-e.pdf.

Koch T. and Harrington A. (1998) Reconceptualizing rigor: the case for reflexivity. *Journal of Advanced Nursing*, **28**, 882–890.

National Health and Medical Research Council (NHMRC) (2007) NHMRC standards and procedures for externally developed guidelines. Retrieved 10 December from: http://www.nhmrc.gov.au/publications/synopses/_files/nh56.pdf. Canberra, ACT: Australian Government.

Northway R. (2000) Disability, nursing research and the importance of reflexivity. *Journal of Advanced Nursing*, **32**, 391–397.

Tashakkori A. and Teddlie C. (eds) (2003) *Handbook of Mixed Methods in Social and Behavioral Research.* Thousand Oaks, California: Sage Publications.

Thurston W. (2006) Methodological congruence in complex and collaborative mixed method projects. *International Journal of Multiple Research Approaches*, **1**, 2–14.

Waldrop D.P. (2007) Caregiver grief in terminal illness and bereavement: a mixed-methods study. *Health and Social Work*, **32**, 197–206.

Wirtz V., Cribb A. and Barber N. (2006) Patient–doctor decision-making about treatment within the consultation – a critical analysis of models. *Social Science and Medicine*, **62**, 116–124.

Does Mixed Methods Constitute a Change in Paradigm?

Tessa Muncey

Learning objectives

After reading this chapter, you will have the knowledge to:

a) Discuss the philosophical debates about mixed methods.
b) Describe pragmatism as an underpinning to mixed methods.
c) Describe the influence of evidence-based practice on design choices.

Introduction

Contemporary health care is facing many competing demands on its resources. This is in response to increases in knowledge, technological and pharmaceutical innovation, together with the rise of the consumer culture which has extended into health care services. With evidence-based decision making guiding the management of health care 'it is incumbent upon healthcare professionals to act collectively to ensure the provision of high quality, cost effective, sociologically and politically conscientious care' (Frank-Stromborg and Olsen 2004: xi). Whilst this may be the consensus amongst health care researchers, the arena in which the evidence is collected is a veritable battlefield. Theoretically, researchers philosophise about the different perspectives that underpin the various methodologies and devise innovative strategies for combining these, 'while at the same time respecting the distinct branches of philosophical thought from which they are derived' (Bowling 2002: 131). However, in practice, rather than quantitative and qualitative research existing as two concepts in the same milieu, to answer different questions in the most pertinent way, a battle for hierarchical dominance exists. Although evidence-based medicine did not set out to confine its sources of evidence to randomised controlled trials (Sackett et al. 1996), nevertheless, they have become the gold standard for research evidence (Belsey and Snell 2003). The consequence of this is to position quantitative methods higher in the hierarchy of best evidence than qualitative methods, with the concomitant impact on what gets more readily funded, published and utilised.

The knowledge claims, strategies of enquiry and methods of data collection within mixed methods approaches in social and behavioural research are well documented (Creswell 2003; Tashakkori and Teddlie 2003). This chapter will consider the implications of these issues within health care research and reinforce the notion that 'different methods have different strengths' dependent on the question under investigation (Morgan in press). Also given the commitment to holistic approaches for tackling health and illness, this chapter will consider whether the hierarchy of knowledge is justified, and whether, in the pursuit of holistic health care practice, the relationship between objectivity and subjectivity is, in fact, a false dichotomy. To set out the context in which these arguments have evolved some consideration of the philosophical issues is required. Although the paradigm wars are considered an historical artefact, there remains an uneasy truce between qualitative and quantitative researchers.

Postwar conflict

Although health care research is dominated by the natural sciences, any analysis of empirical data should be considered in its broader context which may include the environment of health care and the patients' perspective. A consideration of these broader issues has necessitated the adoption of a wider range of methods from the social sciences. This expansion in research methods has led to conflicts about epistemological, ontological and methodological validity and the metaphor of war abounds in the language of the research literature published throughout the 1980s and 1990s. It was around this time that the supporters of quantitative and qualitative approaches in social sciences took up cudgels in opposition. The main protagonists were an elite group of qualitative methodologists who decided to use a set of epistemological and ontological claims to dislodge the dominant position of quantitative research. Rather than promoting the value of qualitative research on its own merits, these advocates created a caricature of quantitative research that they called positivism and then waged a war against it at the level of ontology and epistemology. This resulted in the need for 'lengthy justifications' when selecting a methodology, with precious time wasted arguing about the philosophical underpinnings of other people's research. Are these philosophical underpinnings a help or a hindrance?

On the battle ground were those who claim deductive reasoning, objectivity and generality as the hallmarks of quantitative research, which contrasted diametrically with the inductive, subjective and contextual approach of qualitative research. Gage's (1989) metaphor of paradigm wars was protested by Guba and Lincoln (1994) but whilst they are now considered to be a thing of the past, their legacy remains, particularly in medical research where evidence-based medicine has become synonymous with the randomised controlled trial. What appears to be missing in this struggle, particularly in health care research, is the reason for doing research in the first place. That is, the questions that need answers and the problems that need solutions. The needs of the individual researcher to seek solutions for problems appear neglected in the struggle for funding, getting published in the right journals and the influence of pharmaceutical companies on the health research industry. It could be argued that this contest between so-called opposing sides is actually a civil war. In-fighting between two factions that, if united, would provide a wide repertoire of useful tools in which to produce different types of knowledge to inform practice. Where the kinds of methods you want to use depend upon the kind of knowledge you want to generate. If questions are the central concern, then the next step is not to deny the value of validity but to put it in its right place – as an appropriate standard for judging the use of certain kinds of methods to produce certain kinds of knowledge.

Philosophical disputations

The use of the randomised controlled trial is well established in the canon of medical research but qualitative research drawing on the methodologies of the social sciences and spurred on by postmodernist thinking has also become increasingly prominent, particularly in nursing research; not least because it is able to illuminate behaviour, perceptions and interactions in the complex world of health care. However, despite its utility in exploratory research, the qualitative approach is often given less credibility than quantitative enquiry. The dominance of empiricism in health care research is related to the desire for facts to underpin treatment and intervention decisions.

The caricature for this type of 'truth' in its narrowest sense is positivism, the philosophy of Auguste Comte (1798–1857) who invented the term for his ambitious work, *The Positive Philosophy*, first published in 1830. Comte's (Comte 2000) aim was to provide a systematic survey of all knowledge. Given the size of the enterprise, he limited himself to facts whose truth was unquestionable, whose validity was ensured by the recognised methods of science. Unfortunately, it came to be used rather loosely to describe any discussion of human beings phrased in the language of the natural sciences. The positivists were strongly attracted to the empiricists who believed that the source of true knowledge about the universe is sensory experience, such as what can be seen, heard, felt, tasted, or smelled, or what can be inferred, such as sensory facts. Positivists also found support from the materialists who believed that everything can be understood in terms of the properties of matter and energy. Finally, the positivists had very close ties with the evolutionists. Part of Comte's theory is that civilisation evolves through three stages: the theological, the metaphysical and the positive. This explains the evolutionary theory of society and it is not surprising that Comte's supporters were among the first to support Darwin's theory of biological evolution.

If the acquisition of knowledge, in health care, is seen as dependent on experience then a critical aspect for medical science is the interpretation of experience in everyday understanding. Paradoxically, medicine which purports to adopt a holist stance, follows an empirical approach whilst accepting the Cartesian dualism of the body being divided into mind and matter (Flew 1984). For Descartes (1596–1650) the world was made up of these two incompatible kinds of substance and arguably, until the phenomenon of consciousness and its relationship to physics is better understood, the Cartesian picture is unlikely to lose its hold on the imagination. Bentall (2003) argues that there is a continuing naivety about relationships between biology and psychology and that, as dualisms are so entrenched in our language, it has become almost inevitable, particularly in the arena of mental health, to assume that processes underlying any abnormal behaviour must be attributed to biology or psychology instead of a better understanding of how they interact.

Leaving aside what constitutes knowledge and how it is generated, health care decision makers also have a moral responsibility implicit in the choices that have to be made about which treatments or interventions to select for individuals. Weber (1949) doubted whether extreme rationalist views could ever provide answers to how to live an ethical life. They provide answers to specify how to reach certain goals but cannot say what goals we should strive to reach. In the words of Tolstoy 'science is meaningless because it gives no answer to our question, what shall we do and how shall we live?' (cited in Weber 1958: 143). This is particularly apt as changes to lifestyle are one of the driving forces behind the management of people with long-term conditions in health care.

Paradigms

Since the industrial revolution, science has replaced theology and philosophy as a guiding principle of human existence. This has, without doubt, transformed the world in which we live. The technological triumphs were so remarkable that until recently no one questioned the absolute authority of science in determining the basic strategies of life. In Kuhn's (1962) study of the development of scientific theories and revolutions in science, he observed certain fundamental differences between the social and natural sciences. He noted the disagreements among social scientists concerning the basic nature of legitimate problems and approaches which differed with that of the natural scientists. Whilst social scientists were busy questioning the nature of reality, the practitioners of the physical sciences did not get involved in these controversies. He concluded that the history and philosophy of science as a smooth, logical, increasingly accurate description of the universe leading to the ultimate truth is a distorted and romanticised image of the actual course of events. Rather than the accumulation of data and formulation of ever more accurate theories, science is clearly cyclical with specific stages and characteristic dynamics. Kuhn suggested that the central concept for understanding this was the paradigm.

A paradigm can be defined as 'a shared set of rules and beliefs about how a discipline functions, including what counts as knowledge, how it can be generated and how and by whom it can be generated' (Rolfe 1996: 232). In order to cope with the enormity of the complexity of reality, a scientist must reduce the problem to a workable scale because a consideration of all variables would be unmanageable. Therefore, even in the objective world of science, the scientist brings their own belief system into the study. No paradigm explains all the facts. Indeed, many paradigms can theoretically account for the same set of data. A new and radical theory is never just an addition or increment to existing knowledge. Rules are changed, revision is required to existing assumptions and new thinking must be applied to existing facts and observations. With the publication of Einstein's theory of relativity the ordered rational world of Newtonian physics was cast into doubt, a change which required the rejection of a widely accepted scientific theory. Kuhn (1962) suggested that these revolutions are preceded by a period of conceptual chaos where anomalies are discovered or problems resist the repeated efforts of prominent scientists. When paradigms are accepted they become an accurate picture of reality instead of being seen as a useful model or map.

In the last 300 years western science has been dominated by the Newtonian–Cartesian paradigm. Isaac Newton's (1687) mechanistic view of the universe, developed by physics, became an important criterion of scientific legitimacy in more complex and less developed fields such as the social sciences and medicine. René Descartes' (1596–1650) most significant contribution was the formulation of the absolute dualism between mind and matter resulting in a belief that the material world can be described objectively without reference to the human observer (Cottingham et al. 1991). The legacy of this concept is a serious neglect of a holistic approach to human beings, society and life on this planet. Conveniently forgotten is the role of God in the legacy of these two great thinkers. Both believed that God was an essential element in their world views, but the image of divine intelligence has disappeared from the picture.

One of the still unexplainable events that occurred to dent the power of the Newtonian–Cartesian model was that seemingly unconscious, inert matter became aware of itself and of the surrounding world and consciousness appeared. In the early days of psychology in Wundt's laboratory when the methods of physiology began to be applied to the problems of philosophy, the study of consciousness was recognised as a central concern. William James (1950) objected to this method; he pointed out that sensations are an abstraction we impose on our experiences, they are not an intrinsic part of the experience itself and are subject to continual change, 'experience is remoulding us every moment, and our mental reaction on every given thing is really a resultant of our experience of the whole world up to date' (p. 233–234).

The old science then has been transformative but its essential problems are that it is so different from the way humans behave and experience life. Post Newtonian science embraces a more fluid and relativistic understanding in quantum physics. Unpredictability is a major feature of life and solid boundaries are beneath the superficial appearance plastic and permeable. Unfortunately old science had far more influence than just as a source of new technology. The way that people did scientific thinking was considered to be the model of how thinking should always be done. This intellectual style excluded insights and connections but continues to be the way that health care produces evidence with a strong patient-centred focus. See Box 2.1.

> **Box 2.1 Point to ponder**
>
> The research design, data collection methods and data analysis should all be consistent with the paradigm that underpins a research project. This also applies to mixed methods research.

Hierarchies

Another legacy of Cartesian dualisms is the western propensity to organise everything into a hierarchical structure: man/woman, reason/passion, mind/body, quantitative/qualitative. According to Saussure, the binary opposition is the 'means by which the units of language have value or meaning; each unit is defined against what it is not' (Fogarty 2005). It is fundamentally a structurally derived notion which acknowledges the human inclination to think antagonistically. The desire for a centre generates binary oppositions and Derrida's work illustrates the problematic character of all centres, that all western thought forms binary oppositions where one component of the pair is privileged (Derrida 1978).

This privilege places quantitative research and medicine in a dominant role. In an attempt to establish respectability in their own discourses other professions allied to medicine have moved their 'training' into higher education. This has enabled them to set about acquiring a systematic knowledge base mainly from the established academic disciplines such as the social and natural sciences. Bines (1992) refers to this as technocratic education which Schön (1987) deemed to be unsuitable for practice-based disciplines. In the drive towards evidence-based practice, any practice based on experience and expertise is negated. Practitioners are rarely 'invested with the power and authority to define what counts as research, how it is to be conducted and which in turn determines what constitutes knowledge and truth, and which ultimately reinforces the authority of those in power and the power of those in authority' (Rolfe 1996: 201).

Although current philosophical thinking suggests that all understanding is antecedence – contextual and historic – in order to compete with the dominant force of medicine, other professions allied to medicine have been forced to adopt evidence-based medicine in order to achieve credibility. This is particularly true of nursing which is often seen as task orientated and subservient to medicine, but whose adoption of the social sciences has enabled a discrete body of knowledge to develop that reflects both the art and science of the discipline (Muncey 2006). Practitioners of health care grapple with the schism between theory and practice and many see beyond the between quantitative and qualitative dichotomy and advocate what Bond (1993) calls 'method-ological pluralism and pragmatism'. Chapman (1991) goes further to suggest that the positivist and interpretive schools are in fact just two different approaches to data collection and analysis. The dominance of medicine is still apparent, although evidence-based medicine was sup-posed to impact on clinical practice and cost effectiveness, improve patient outcomes and move decision making away from the role of expert to one of evidence.

Individualism

No consideration of appropriate methods can be divorced from the objects or subjects of study. The western world has embraced the pursuit of individualism and this has placed greater responsibility on the individual to take responsibility for their own health (Muncey and Parker 2002). It is at the level of the individual that decisions are made about treatments and interventions but paradoxically research trials require large populations which ignore the individual perspective. This contradiction may be responsible for the failure of compliance with health care advice as individuals' beliefs and choices are left out of the equation. The common denominator in any studies of people and health care is the body. Arguably every aspect of our lives is embodied and one of the important factors to consider in any health care research is the 'changing nature of the disease burden', for example amongst many other things, the impact of chronic illness, demonstrating that 'biophysical changes have significant social consequences' (Nettleton and Watson 1998: 5). Shilling (2003) argues that although the body has a material, biological base this is altered and modified within different social constructs. So the subjective experience of health and disease cannot be separated from the attempts to explain it objectively.

Pragmatism

Pragmatists are accused of the abandonment of traditional standards of objectivity, truth and rationality. However, what James (1995: 77) questions is that 'grant an idea to be true, what concrete difference will its being true make in anyone's actual life? How will the truth be realised? What experiences will be different from those which would obtain if the belief were false? What, in short, is the truth's cash-value in experiential terms?' To James (1995: 77) 'truth is not a stagnant prop-erty inherent in it. Truth happens to an idea.' Pragmatists accept the problem-solving function of human beliefs. All human activity arises from our need to solve problems. A true statement or belief is one that is useful in solving a problem.

Whilst in problem solving a statement or belief is true when it corresponds to the facts, there may be statements that we believe to be true for which there are no facts. It is only possible to check facts by making observations or meeting empirical criteria for knowledge of the external, observable world.

One objection to this is that it is inadequate as a criterion for non-empirical statements. In contrast a coherence theory of truth is defined by reference to the reasons we have for believing something to be true. Therefore a particular belief may be true when it is part of a coherent set of mutually supported beliefs. Therefore pragmatically 'truth' is better replaced with 'efficacy' or just plain effectiveness.

The fallacy of a false dichotomy arises when the premise of an argument presents us with a choice between two alternatives and presumes that they are exhaustive, or exclusive, or both, when in fact they are not. Avis (2003) argues that Quine (1953) disposed of positivism with the suggestions that verificationism depended on two unsustainable assumptions. Firstly by reductionism, where all experience must be reduced to empirical evidence provided by the senses. Secondly, the distinction between synthetic truths, true because of the way the world is, and analytic truths, true because of the meanings of the terms they contain. By separating theory and evidence Avis suggests that positivism was doomed and furthermore qualitative methodology is counter-productive because it hinders critical reflection on the relationship between methodological theory and empirical evidence. In a holistic view of knowledge, which health care purports to draw on, are there really any fundamental epistemological differences between empirical methods and those concerned with factual matters or subjective human experience? See Box 2.2.

Box 2.2 Point to ponder

Fundamental to pragmatism is the belief that the research questions should be the impetus for choosing research design not a method or a paradigm.

Researching evidence for health

There is no disputing that research is seen as an important step in improving the health and well-being of the population and to provide modern, effective health and social care services. It provides the important link to inform and develop high-quality evidence-based care for the public (Mant et al. 2004; Majeed 2005). In the UK a number of government publications indicate a need to improve the way research is conducted to put the UK at the forefront of research development and innovation (Department of Health 2000a & b, 2005b, 2006). To support changes in research and development the UK Clinical Research Collaboration (UKCRC) was created with the ultimate goal of promoting an extensive and sustained increase in the research workforce (Walport 2005; Finch 2007).

Implicit in this drive to increase the research workforce is the capacity to produce evidence that supports clinical decision making and makes effective use of resources whilst still maintaining a patient-centred approach. Increasing public expectations and demographic changes have combined with political change and reform to have a profound effect on the provision of health care. Government policy since 1998 in the UK has consistently sought to increase patient involvement in health care decision making (Department of Health 2005a) and promotion of a key role for primary care physicians (Department of Health 2004) in commissioning health care provision. A patient-centred approach involves a systematic history-taking together with consideration of patients' ideas, knowledge, beliefs and expectations (Alder et al. 2004). There is evidence of improved satisfaction among patients who experience a patient-centred approach (Lewin et al. 2001; Little et al. 2001; Stewart 2001), while failure to elicit and respond empathically to beliefs and expectations has been found to be associated with decreased satisfaction and reduced compliance (Tuckett et al. 1985; Haywood et al. 2006; Chio et al. 2008). See Box 2.3.

Box 2.3 Research in action

In a study of the expectations of prescriptions, ethnicity, age, gender, symptoms, prescription charge status, appointment booking and day of the week were all issues that were deemed to make a difference to patient attitudes (Britten et al. 2002). Similarly, in their study examining patients' expectations of tests, referrals and medications in primary care visits, Peck et al. (2004) identified that the most important factor in determining satisfaction concerned the way the patient was managed in the patient–physician relationship rather than the meeting of technical expectations such as referrals or diagnostic tests.

Evidence-based medicine

In considering the position of mixed methods in health care research it is impossible to ignore the current preoccupation with evidence-based medicine. Evidence-based medicine establishes a hierarchy of knowledge. Different types of clinical evidence are categorised and ranked according to the strength of their freedom from bias, making 'clinical research into the accuracy and precision of diagnostic tests . . . the power of prognostic markers, and the efficacy and safety of therapeutic, rehabilitative, and preventive regimens' the focus (Sackett et al. 1996: 71). In addition to the false dichotomy of subjectivity and objectivity this hierarchy may not provide the best evidence. The research question should be the most important feature impacting on the research design, which results in the choice of either quantitative or qualitative approaches or mixed approaches where appropriate.

The primary purpose of any health care system should be to achieve the greatest possible improvement in the physical and mental health of the population. Although historically, testing the efficacy of medical interventions has always existed, by the end of the twentieth century this had evolved to impact on all fields of health care and policy. The term 'evidence-based medicine' first appeared in the medical literature in 1992 (Guyatt et al. 1992). What evidence-based medicine attempts to do is apply the standards of evidence gained from the scientific method to certain aspects of medical practice and apply judgements to the quality of that evidence.

Evidence-based medicine is defined as 'the conscientious, explicit and judicious use of current best evidence in making decisions about the care of individual patients. The practice of evidence-based medicine means integrating individual clinical expertise with the best available external clinical evidence from systematic research' (Sackett et al. 1996: 71). The advent of evidence-based medicine has witnessed the downgrading of the evidence provided by the social sciences to the extent where it is considered the lowest level of evidence in an evidence-based hierarchy.

This hierarchy may have the added influence of reinforcing the theory–practice gap. Knowledge derived from clinical research may not be directly applicable to individual patients 'as the knowledge gained from clinical research does not directly answer the primary clinical question of what is best for the patient at hand' (Tonelli 2001: 1435). Tonelli (2001) further argues that empirical evidence and clinical experience differ in kind, not in degree, and do not belong on a graded hierarchy. This lack of applicability has implications for the claim that randomised controlled trials alone are the gold standard of evidence.

Randomised controlled trials: a gold standard?

Do randomised controlled trials actually do what they claim to do? Context would appear to be an important consideration. There are at least two ways for questioning randomised controlled trials as a false gold standard. Firstly: are randomised controlled trials the best way to do any kind of research? We believe their value is much greater for some purposes than others. Randomised controlled trials are important for the development of well verified, objective, reducible research but we question their usefulness for exploratory research.

A second criticism is that randomised controlled trials may have similar results in the 'real' world as they do in the original trial. This is partly because too much emphasis may be placed on internal validity to the extend that external validity is compromised or too little attention is paid to 'ecological validity' (Lincoln and Guba 1985). In other words, randomised controlled trials too often ignore the complexity of the context in which ill-health and its management occurs. Health care problems are not simply reducible to the act of taking a pill to regulate a strictly biological process, which alludes to the fundamental analogy of a double-blind, placebo randomised controlled trial as a gold standard. See Box 2.4.

Box 2.4 Point to ponder

When levels of evidence are presented in a hierarchical list, systematic reviews of randomised controlled trials are always considered the strongest level of evidence. Expert opinion is always located at the furthest point from randomised controlled trials and is considered the weakest level of evidence.

Many of the health care problems experienced by individuals today do not fit that 'one pill for one problem' model. Instead, they are more likely to be complex, chronic conditions that involve equally complex approaches to management regimes which frequently involve behaviour change. We believe trying to treat those kinds of problems in a context-free fashion is ludicrous, and trying to set up a series of randomised controlled trials that would modify the relevant contextual factors one at a time would be a fool's errand. See Box 2.5.

Box 2.5 Research in action

A very large randomised controlled trial evaluated the use of existing medications for the management of a common chronic condition (Morgan 2007). The study incorporated qualitative focus groups with doctors who were involved in the trial. Findings indicated that these doctors perceived that:

- Inclusion and exclusion criteria often led to trials where the patients being tested did not match the larger population of patients that the doctors saw in actual practice.
- One specific result of these exclusion criteria was that it greatly reduced the number of older patients who were eligible, due to the common presence of multiple chronic conditions among older patients.
- The quality of care provided to patients in trials did not match routine practice.
- The patients' participation in the trial meant that they received a much higher level of routine monitoring than other patients.

Competing perspectives of health and disease

Part of the reason for a wide range of research tools lies in the complexity of the nature of the subject area. The study of health and disease ranges from the macro level of populations right down to the micro level of microbiology whilst most practice deals with individuals. Add environmental issues to the mix and the difficulties of providing useful evidence to inform practice are clear. The dominant model of disease in the western hemisphere is the bio-medical model based on the Cartesian philosophy of the body as a machine. Treatments for the disease that results from malfunctioning of the body tend to ignore the subjective experience of this malfunction. The mind as opposed to the brain is not considered to cause disease although psychological sequelae of disease may occur. Illness is the experience of having a disease. Research in health care in the west has been dominated by scientific methods but given the complexity of holistic medicine, it would appear that drawing on the most appropriate methods and mixing them where appropriate would provide the sophisticated range of evidence on which to base practice.

Conclusion

So does mixing methods constitute a change in paradigm? Is the dichotomy between subjective and objective views of the world a false one? Might the civil war not actually be a skirmish amongst opposing gangs in the same city? It could be argued, as Rose (1991) does very eloquently in *Governing the Soul*, that the autonomy of self is a delusion with subjectivity controlled by experts. Whilst citizens of liberal democracies appear to shape their lives 'it is possible to govern subjectivity according to norms and criteria that ground their authority in an esoteric but objective knowledge' (Rose 1991: 9).

Subjectivity implies that everybody has a different world view, that somehow we can separate ourselves from 'out there' and produce a view that is distinct from the objective world of science. However, in the last several hundred years the sense of self, it could be argued, has evolved amidst the development of many hypothetical constructs such as personality, memory, intelligence, perception, quality of life to name a few. These concepts have been carefully contrived by social scientists, using empiricist and materialist approaches as well as constructivist ones, and are now part of our 'unexamined assumptions' about who we are and are implicit features of our sense of self, making it virtually impossible to say where the objective world stops and the subjective view begins. So whilst many would argue about the nature of memory, its uses, how it works and its structure, nobody appears to question whether memory exists at all. Likewise within the medical model arguments arise over treatments and compliance and the extent to which genetics or environment affect the body most, but there is generally little disagreement that the body works by homeostasis.

However, it is possible that the health care world is in what Kuhn described as a 'pre paradigm period' (Kuhn 1970: 187). Bloom (2000: xii–xiii) describes this as the holistic revolution, in which the 'very nature of the post-modern global village – the contemporary way of researching, perceiving and interpreting – is that people will seek information as widely as possible'. That is, a world where the unanswered questions about consciousness find answers, and spirituality and soul return from their neglected position in the wonder and meaning of what it is to be a human being. This is evidenced by the dramatic rise in the popularity of alternative medical approaches during the 1990s, when 42% (some 83 million) of adult Americans, used one or more alternative therapies (Eisenberg et al. 1998). Many of these therapies are outside the usual scientific world view and perhaps the shift in paradigm will occur when the health disciplines realise that more daring alternatives of investigation are needed.

A real paradigm shift will have occurred when the unconscious mind is seen as an integral aspect of scientific thinking. The revolution to unite the mind–body continuum has started and can be seen in Pert's (1997) 'Molecules of emotion' where she describes an information network which links mind and body in a way previously considered impossible and unthinkable. It is evident in the huge popularity of Chopra's (1990) writing about a mind–body approach to cancer. Also in *Beyond the Brain*, Grof (1985) poses a new model of the human psyche that has been challenging the adequacy of the scientific world for some decades. When this type of thinking becomes 'normal science' then a paradigm change will have occurred. In the meantime the false dichotomy of objective/subjective should be viewed for what it is, two ends of the same spectrum. Heisenberg (1955) suggested that instead of looking for and finding objective qualities when examining nature and the universe 'man encounters himself'. To which Wolfgang Pauli adds by creating a parallel between our investigation of outer objects, with a psychological investigation of the inner origin of our scientific concepts, we will achieve a 'oneness' between the physical and the psychological spheres and the quantitative and qualitative aspects of reality (cited in Franz 1978). Until a unifying paradigm is accepted the antagonistic qualities of the current binary opposition could be removed and both valued for what they do well, namely providing answers to different types of questions, then the researchers can get on with the refining of their craft in the pursuit of benefiting people's health care needs. This is entirely in keeping with the pragmatist suggestion 'that knowledge, rather than mirroring an outer world, is about making a difference . . . in which the pursuit of knowledge goes hand in hand with a responsibility to bring about change' (Baert 2005: 169).

References

Alder B., Porter M., Abraham C. and van Teijlingen E. (2004) *Psychology and Sociology Applied to Medicine.* London: Churchill Livingstone.

Avis M. (2003) Pearls, pith and provocation. Do we need methodological theory to do qualitative research? *Qualitative Health Research*, **13**, 995–1004.

Baert P. (2005) *Philosophy of the Social Sciences.* Cambridge: Polity Press.

Belsey J. and Snell T. (2003) What is evidence-based medicine? Hayward Group PLC. Accessed 1 April 2008 at www.evidence-based-medicine.co.uk/ebmfiles/Whatisebm.pdf.

Bentall R.P. (2003) *Madness Explained: Psychosis and Human Nature.* London: Penguin.

Bines H. (1992) Issues in course design. In Bines H. and Watson D. (eds.) *Developing Professional Education*, pp. 11–26. Buckingham: Open University Press.

Bloom W. (ed.) (2000) *Holistic Revolution: The Essential New Age Reader.* London: Penguin Books.

Bond S. (1993) Experimental research in nursing: necessary but not sufficient. In Kitson A. (ed.) *Nursing: Art and Science.* London: Chapman and Hall.

Bowling A. (2002) *Research Methods in Health: Investigating Health and Health Services.* Maidenhead: Open University Press.

Britten N., Ukoumunne O. and Boulton M. (2002) Patients' attitudes to medicines and expectations for prescriptions. *Health Expectations*, **5**, 256–269.

Chapman J. (1991) Research – what it is and what it is not. In Perry A. and Jolley M. (eds.) *Nursing: A Knowledge Base for Practice.* London: Edward Arnold.

Chio A., Montuschi A., Cammarosano S., Mercanti D., Cavallo E., Illardi A. et al. (2008) ALS patients' and caregivers' communication preferences and information seeking behaviour. *European Journal of Neurology*, **15**, 55–60.

Chopra D. (1990) *Quantum Healing: Exploring the Frontiers of Mind Body Medicine.* New York: Bantum Books.

Comte A. (2000) *The Positive Philosophy.* Kitchener, Ontario: Batoche Books.

Cottingham J., Stoothoff R. and Murdoch D. (eds.) (1991) *The Philosophical Writings of Descartes.* Cambridge: Cambridge University Press.

Creswell J.W. (2003) *Research Design: Qualitative, Quantitative and Mixed Methods Approaches.* London: Sage Publications.

Department of Health (2000a) *Research and Development for a First Class Service: R&D Funding in the New NHS.* London: DOH.

Department of Health (2000b) *Towards a Strategy for Nursing Research and Development – Proposals for Action.* London: DOH.

Department of Health (2004) *Practice Based Commissioning: Promoting Clinical Engagement.* London: DOH.

Department of Health (2005a) *Creating a Patient-led NHS: Delivering the NHS Improvement Plan.* London: DOH.

Department of Health (2005b) *Research Governance Framework for Health and Social Care*, 2nd edition. London: DOH.

Department of Health (2006) *Best Research for Best Health: A New National Health Research Strategy.* London: DOH.

Derrida J. (1978) *Writing and Difference.* London: Routledge and Kegan Paul.

Eisenberg D.M., Davis R.B., Ettner S.L., Scott Appel M., Wilkey S., Van Rompay M. et al. (1998) Trends in alternative medicine use in the United States, 1990–1997. *Journal of the American Medical Association*, **280**, 1569–1575.

Finch J. (2007) *Developing the Best Research Professionals.* Report of the UKCRC Sub Committee for Nurses in Clinical Research (Workforce). UK Clinical Research Collaboration.

Flew A. (ed.) (1984) *A Dictionary of Philosophy.* London: Pan Books.

Fogarty S. (2005) Binary Oppositions. *The Literary Encyclopaedia.* Accessed 1 April 2008, www.litencyc.com/php/stopics.php?rec=true&UID=122.

Frank-Stromborg M. and Olsen S.J. (2004) *Instruments for Clinical Health-care Research.* London: Jones and Bartlett Publishers.

Franz M.-L. (1978) Science and the unconscious. In Jung C. (ed.) *Man and his Symbols*, pp. 375–388. London: Picador.

Gage N. (1989) The paradigm wars and their aftermath: a 'historical' sketch of research and teaching since 1989. *Educational Researcher*, **18**, 4–10.

Grof S. (1985) *Beyond the Brain: Birth, Death and Transcendence in Psychotherapy.* New York: State University of New York.

Guba E.G. and Lincoln Y.S. (1994) Competing paradigms in qualitative research. In Denzin N.K. and Lincoln Y.S. (eds.) *Handbook of Qualitative Research*, pp. 105–117. Thousand Oaks, CA: Sage.

Guyatt G., Cairns J. and Churchill D. (1992) Evidence-based medicine. A new approach to teaching the practice of medicine. *Journal of the American Medical Association*, **268**, 2420–2425.

Haywood K., Marshall S. and Fitzpatrick R. (2006) Patient participation in the consultation process: a structured review of intervention strategies. *Patient Education and Counselling*, **63**, 12–23.

Heisenberg W. (1955) The development of the interpretation of the quantum theory. In Pauli W. (ed.) *Niels Bohr and the Development of Physics. Essays Dedicated to Niels Bohr on the Occasion of his Seventieth Birthday*, pp. 12–29. New York: McGraw Hill.

James W. (1950) *The Principles of Psychology.* New York: Dover Publications.

James W. (1995) *Pragmatism.* New York: Dover Publications.

Kuhn T. (1962) *The Structure of Scientific Revolutions.* Chicago: University of Chicago Press.

Kuhn T. (1970) *The Structure of Scientific Revolutions*, 2nd edition. Chicago: University of Chicago Press.

Lewin S., Skea Z., Entwhistle V., Zwarenstein M. and Dick J. (2001) Interventions for providers to promote a patient-centred approach to clinical consultations. *Cochrane Database of Systematic Reviews*, Issue 4. Art. No. CD003267. DOI: 10.1002/14651858.CD003267.

Lincoln Y.S. and Guba E.G. (1985) *Naturalistic Inquiry.* Newbury Park CA: Sage.

Little P., Everett H. and Williamson I. (2001) Preferences of patients for patient-centred approach to consultation in primary care: observational study. *British Medical Journal*, **322**, 468–472.

Majeed A. (2005) Primary care trusts and primary care research. *British Medical Journal*, **330**, 56–57.

Mant D., DelMar C., Glasziou P., Knottnerus A., Wallace P. and van Weel C. (2004) The state of primary care research. *Lancet*, **364**, 1004–1006.

Morgan D.L. (2007) Research in action. Personal communication.

Morgan D.L. (Forthcoming) *Integrating Qualitative and Quantitative Methods: A Pragmatic Approach.* Thousand Oaks, CA: Sage.

Muncey T. (2006) Mixing art and science: a bridge over troubled waters or a bridge too far? *Journal of Research in Nursing*, **11**, 223–233.

Muncey T. and Parker A. (eds.) (2002) *Chronic Disease Management: A Practical Guide.* Basingstoke: Palgrave.

Nettleton S. and Watson J. (1998) Introduction. In Nettleton S. and Watson J. (eds.) *The Body in Everyday Life*, pp. 1–24. London: Routledge.

Newton I. (1687) *Philosophiæ Naturalis Principia Mathematica.* London: Joseph Streater for the Royal Society, London.

Peck M., Ubel P., Debra L., Roter D., Goold S., Asch D. et al. (2004) Do unmet expectations for specific test, referrals and new medications reduce patients' satisfaction? *Journal of General Internal Medicine,* **19**, 1080–1087.

Pert C. (1997) Psychoneuroimmunology; molecules of emotion. In Bloom W. (ed.) *Holistic Revolution: The Essential New Age Reader.* London: Penguin Books.

Quine W. (1953) *From a Logical Point of View.* Cambridge, MA: Harvard University Press.

Rolfe G. (1996) *Closing the Theory–Practice Gap: A New Paradigm for Nursing.* Oxford: Butterworth Heinnemann.

Rose N. (1991) *Governing the Soul: The Shaping of the Private Self.* London: Routledge.

Sackett D.L., Rosenberg W.M., Muir Gray J., Haynes R.B. and Richardson W.S. (1996) Editorial. *British Medical Journal,* **312**, 71–72.

Schön D. (1987) *Educating the Reflective Practitioner.* San Francisco: Jossey-Bass.

Shilling C. (2003) *The Body and Social Theory.* London: Sage Publications.

Stewart M. (2001) Towards a global definition of patient centred care. *British Medical Journal,* **322**, 444–445.

Tashakkori A. and Teddlie C. (2003) *Handbook of Mixed Methods in Social and Behavioral Research.* Thousand Oaks, CA: Sage.

Tonelli M. (2001) The limits of evidence based medicine. *Respiratory Care,* **46**, 1435–1440.

Tuckett D., Boulton M., Oslen C. and Williams A. (1985) *Meeting Between Experts: an Approach to Sharing Ideas in Medical Consultation.* London: Tavistock Publishers.

Walport M. (2005) *Medically Qualified and Dentally Qualified Academic Staff: Recommendations for Training the Researchers and Educators of the Future.* Report of the Academic Careers Sub Committee of Modernising Medical Careers and the UK Clinical Research Collaboration. UKCRC.

Weber M. (1949) *The Methodology of the Social Sciences.* Illinois: Free Press.

Weber M. (1958) *From Max Weber.* New York: Oxford University Press.

Designs for Mixed Methods Research

Thilo Kroll and Melinda Neri

Learning objectives

The purpose of this chapter is to examine design considerations when planning mixed methods studies. After reading this chapter you will have the knowledge to:

a) Understand the importance of clearly linking the research design to the purpose and question of the study.
b) Locate mixed methods designs in the context of designing research that is context- and population-sensitive.
c) Identify various mixed methods design types and related sampling strategies.
d) Describe key features of commonly used mixed methods research designs.
e) Understand the rationale for selecting particular mixed methods designs.
f) Identify design-specific methods that can be used to answer research questions.

Introduction

A wide variety of mixed methods designs has been described in the literature. This stems from the potential for creativity on the part of researchers using this approach. Whilst over 40 designs have been

categorised (Tashakkori and Teddlie 2003), these can be reduced to a
few core designs with signature features that clearly distinguish them
from one another. In this chapter the characteristics of the common
mixed method designs are discussed and the questions that researchers
need to consider when using these designs are explored.

The reader is cautioned to carefully consider the rationale for their
use of a mixed methods design. There are circumstances where traditional homogeneous research designs may be preferable. Even when
the rationale for mixed methods research designs is sound there may
be multiple reasons why investigators will choose traditional design
approaches. These include a lack of expertise or resources within
the research team, stakeholder priorities and dissemination issues
(Table 3.1).

Table 3.1 Reasons for choosing mixed methods rather than 'traditional' designs.

Consideration	Explanation
Research purpose	• The research purpose and research questions require a combination of qualitative and quantitative methods. • Research questions can be formulated to either provide testable results (quantitative) or to describe and characterise a phenomenon of interest (qualitative) but individually they do not address the primary purpose of the study. • There is insufficient information available in the literature and there is a need for exploratory research.
Research expertise	• A team that has expertise in qualitative and quantitative research methods and how to combine them for mixed methods research can be found and are willing to work together collaboratively.
Resources	• There is funding available to conduct a multiphase, multimethod study.
Stakeholder priorities	• Policymakers want detailed coverage of the problem including the extent (quantitative) or nature (qualitative) of a problem and how they are interrelated.
Dissemination	• Journal accepts mixed methods research papers.

Research purpose and design

Research design is concerned with transforming research questions into a framework of strategies and methods that will enable the investigator to systematically answer these questions. The specific strategies and methods used in conducting the research depend on how the research question is formulated. A mixed methods study may have an overarching question that encompasses all aspects of the study, or there may be subquestions which separately guide the qualitative and quantitative components of the data collection.

'Designing' research is not simply a process of assembling an array of data collection methods, but rather should be a carefully selected and systematically applied process. Building a house may serve as an analogy. It is not sufficient to acquire all the raw materials needed to build the foundation, erect the frame, construct the walls and install the appliances. The design process requires careful planning of every step in the process, from calculating static to determining how to wire cables and ensuring that doors have sufficient space to open and close. Good design does not only necessitate relevant expertise, it also ensures that timelines are met, and that tasks are undertaken in a logical sequence. For example, the floor will not be put into your new house before the walls are dry.

'Design deals primarily with aims, purposes, intentions and plans within the practical constraints of location, time, money and availability of staff. It is also very much about style, the architect's own preferences and ideas (whether innovative or solidly traditional) and the stylistic preferences of those who pay for the work and have to live with the finished results' (Hakim 1987: 1). In other words, the research design links a research purpose or question to an appropriate method of data collection and a set of specific outcomes. Newman et al. (2003) have devised a typology of research purposes in the social sciences. These include: 1) prediction, 2) adding to knowledge base, 3) personal, social, institutional and/or organisational impact, 4) measurement of change, 5) understanding complex phenomena, 6) testing of new ideas, 7) generation of new ideas, 8) inform constituencies, 9) examine the past. All of these can be achieved within the context of mixed methods research design.

General design elements

As has been addressed in Chapter 2, different paradigms underpin the way that researchers' believe 'knowledge' or 'evidence' can be uncovered or produced. This has immediate implications for the design of mixed methods research. The debate continues whether seemingly different scientific 'world views' are compatible, or not, and to what degree paradigmatic views necessitate design 'purity'. Mixed methods researchers accept that it is possible to combine qualitative and quantitative methods, but maintain congruence with their respective paradigms.

Regardless of specific research orientation, most research studies follow the same general framework, consisting of the elements listed in Table 3.2. Answering the questions in the right-hand column will guide the researcher towards the design options most appropriate for answering their particular research questions.

Planning a mixed methods study

In mixed methods research, quantitative and qualitative methods are combined in the context of one study. While it is important to understand what other terms are in use to describe the combined use of qualitative and quantitative methods, it is equally critical to determine what does not represent a mixed methods study. We need to distinguish studies that simply combine multiple methods in the data collection or multi-informant studies from mixed methods designs. For example, the use of a questionnaire that contains rating scales, categorical answers, as well as open-ended questions, does not automatically constitute a mixed methods study. Similarly, collecting information from different sources, such as a systematic literature review and key informant interviews, does not automatically indicate a mixed methods approach. For the research to be considered a true mixed methods study, there must be genuine 'integration of the data at one or more stages in the process of research' (Creswell et al. 2003: 212).

For example, a researcher may conduct a study of that employs in-depth interviews with general practitioners, family members of people with learning disabilities and individuals with learning disabilities to examine factors that prevent or facilitate access to general health care services for people with learning disabilities. The study results may lead to findings that show that a range of personal, economic, social and environmental factors impede access to services in complex ways. The results may be an impetus to the researcher to explore further issues from the original study, such as determining the magnitude of the problem with access to dental services for persons with a disability. The nursing researcher may collaborate with a professor in dentistry and a sociologist and the new study design may target a random selection of dental practices in the country and use an online survey format

Table 3.2 Research design elements.

Design element	Questions to answer
Purpose and relevance	• Why is this research necessary? • What knowledge will be derived from this research? • Is the primary purpose to describe, explore, understand, examine, evaluate or test a phenomenon of interest? • Are there multiple purposes for conducting the study?
Theoretical orientation	• Will the study be conducted and analysed within a grounded theory, ethnographic, phenomenological or postpositivist quantitative or pragmatic framework?
Research questions	• Does the research question imply a comparison with a different group? • Does the research question imply magnitude, degree, frequency? • Does the research question imply description, contextualisation and understanding from a particular perspective? • Does the research question require a combination of all of the above?
Sampling strategy	• Will the sampling be based on a random, selective, purposive or convenience process? or, • Will the sampling require a combination of random and non-random strategies?
Methods of investigation	• Will interviews, questionnaires, observations, focus groups or numeric scales and tests be used to answer the research question? or, • Will a combination of data collection methods be used to answer the research question?
Methods of analysis	• Will qualitative or quantitative (statistical) methods of analyses be employed separately to answer the research question? or, • Will integrated methods of data analyses be employed?

for data collection. Despite the fact that this second quantitative study has emerged from the first qualitative one it is not a mixed methods study, as the studies were conducted independently, focusing on different research problems and questions and the findings are not integrated.

Having identified that the study will meet the criteria to be defined as mixed methods research the researcher must choose the design. This is a critical first step and careful attention has to be paid to various planning steps to turn the design into a feasible study. Among the first questions to ask are: 1) Is a mixed methods design appropriate?, and 2) Is a mixed methods design needed? These two questions differ in that the first seeks to establish the scientific appropriateness of a mixed methods design approach. It asks whether the research question as it is formulated can be best answered with mixed methods. The second question examines whether a comprehensive and costly approach such as mixed methods is really needed and whether enough knowledge may already exist in the scientific literature (for example, sufficient quantitative information about the magnitude of an access to care issue) that would suggest a different design choice (for example, a qualitative in-depth study to build a theory about why access difficulties occur).

Effectively designing mixed methods studies not only requires adequate resources (budget, time, software) and expertise (researchers trained in qualitative and quantitative methods and integration of data from both methods) but also the ability to systematically map out the research process (aims, priority, sequence and integration of study parts). Frequently, students are intrigued by the promise they see in mixed methods research. However, they often fail to appreciate the resource implications and expertise required for the conduct of such projects. Additional considerations for research students are discussed in Chapter 12. Some authors have recently discussed the potential for mixed methods designs to be used in multiyear research and development projects involving multiple iterative qualitative and quantitative phases (Schensul et al. 2006; Nastasi et al. 2007) (Box 3.1). In these complex research studies, formative or exploratory research phases are followed by confirmatory and explanatory research phases.

Box 3.1 Research in action

A Sri Lanka Mental Health Promotion Project (SLMHPP) (Nastasi et al. 2007) used a combination of research methods, including focus groups, individual in-depth interviews, key-informant interviews, participant observation, archival material, cultural and historical literature, popular mental health literature and media as well as secondary analyses of existing qualitative and quantitative data to develop culture-specific theory and quantitative psychological self and teacher report measures. The authors contend that 'this mixed methods approach to scale development yielded insights to Sri Lankan youth culture that could not have been obtained with singular approaches' (Nastasi et al. 2007: 174).

Considerations for choosing a mixed methods design

When discussing mixed methods research designs, many authors appear to ignore traditional design features in health and social science research. Robson (2002) distinguishes between 'fixed' and 'flexible' designs. The former is theory-driven and research is conducted to test and hopefully confirm the researcher's theory and hypotheses. Research is mostly conducted under 'controlled' conditions. Flexible designs are mostly 'exploratory' in nature with less control over variables that produce the findings. The strength of mixed methods designs is to balance flexibility of qualitative exploration with the fixed characteristics of theoretical grounding and hypothesis-testing inherent to many quantitative approaches. Mixed methods designs systematically and purposefully combine fixed and flexible design components. The six primary purposes that guide mixed methods research designs are presented in Chapter 4.

Several authors have attempted to provide a classification of the various mixed methods designs (Creswell et al. 2003). While the plethora of terms and designs described in the literature can be confusing, it is important to focus on the research aim and to choose the design most appropriate to answer it. It is important to note that there is currently no standard nomenclature of designs for mixed methods research. Therefore, whilst the most popular design names have been used here, some authors may use slightly different names to describe these designs in their work.

Creswell (2003) proposes four questions that must be addressed by the researcher during the planning stage of mixed methods research:

- In what *sequence* will the qualitative and quantitative data collection be implemented?
- What relative *priority* will be given to the qualitative and quantitative data collection and analysis?
- At what stage of the project will the qualitative and quantitative data be *integrated*?
- Will an overall *theoretical perspective* be used to guide the study?

Implementation sequence

Qualitative and quantitative data can be collected either sequentially or concurrently. In sequential studies one data collection methods follows after the other, whereas, in concurrent studies, the qualitative and quantitative data are collected at the same time. The decision about the implementation sequence is determined by the nature of the research question and the rationale for collecting each dataset. For example, when interviews are intended to provide insight into survey findings they are generally conducted subsequent to the analysis of the survey data (sequentially). However, when qualitative and quantitative data are being collected for confirmation it may be possible to collect the data at the same time (concurrently).

Priority

Another consideration for choosing a design is whether one of the methods (qualitative or quantitative) will have priority or greater emphasis than the other in the study. In other words, priority refers to the relative weight assigned to the qualitative and quantitative research components (Kroll et al. 2005). In exploratory studies, where the concepts, variables and relationships among them are mostly unclear, greater priority is often assigned to qualitative elements that uncover the 'pool' of variables and relationships among them that may be subsequently studied quantitatively. On the other hand, in explanatory research where qualitative research is mostly used to substantiate findings generated in a population-level survey, priority is mostly assigned to the quantitative component. Figure 3.1 depicts the various combinations of implementation and priority that can inform mixed methods designs.

Integration

Perhaps the most important, but least discussed, characteristic of mixed methods research is the 'mixing' of qualitative and quantitative com-

| | | Implementation sequence | |
		Concurrent	Sequential
Priority	**Equal status**	QUAL + QUANT	QUANT → QUAL QUAL → QUANT
	Dominant status	QUAL + quant QUANT + qual	QUAL → quant qual → QUANT QUANT → qual quant → QUAL

+ = concurrent; → = sequential; quant/QUANT = quantitative; qual/QUAL = qualitative; QUANT/QUAL = dominant phase.

Figure 3.1 Mixed method design matrix (Andrew and Halcomb 2007). Reprinted with permission from eContent Management Pty Ltd. Adapted from Creswell et al. 2003; Johnson & Onwuegbuzie 2004; Morgon 1998; Morse 2003.

ponents. True mixed methods designs include a purposeful integration of qualitative and quantitative methods. Integration can occur at various stages of the research process. Integration preferably happens during the data collection, data analysis and/or data interpretation phases but it may also occur in the discussion section of a report/ thesis/journal article. The decision on when and how to integrate the data relates back to the research question, including how it is formulated and whether secondary questions have been stated. It is critical that researchers set out with a clear idea how the different data components inform one another and how they provide distinctive answers to the research questions. Integration must never be an 'afterthought' in that researchers blindly embark on a journey of data collection and then try to make sense of the process. Integration is, in many ways, the pivotal point of mixed methods studies. It is important that researchers reporting mixed methods studies clearly articulate the strategies that have been used to achieve integration to both allow the reader to critique the study and contribute to the scholarly discourse regarding the method.

Theoretical perspective

Mixed methods studies may be underpinned by a theoretical perspective that influences the selection of a particular research design and shapes the research process (Creswell 2003). Theoretical perspectives, such as formalised empirical theories (for example, social cognitive theory (Bandura 1997)), epistemological positions (for example, phenomenology, feminism), social theories (for example, social model of disability (Priestley 2003)), theoretical and practical views about the conduct of research (for example, community-based participatory research (Minkler and Wallerstein 2003)) or theoretical propositions with regard to socio-economic, cultural or lifestyle factors could all be used in varying degrees. Mixed methods designs that are guided by theoretical perspectives are often referred to as transformative designs.

Research designs for mixed methods research

Following consideration of the sequence of data collection, relative priority, process of integration and presence of a theoretical perspective, six primary research designs can be identified (Table 3.3). These designs are divided into two subgroups based on their implementation sequence. The sequential designs include sequential exploratory,

Table 3.3 Mixed methods designs. Creswell et al. (2003) in Tashakkori A. and Teddlie C. (eds.) *Handbook of Mixed Methods in Social and Behavioral Research*, p. 224. Thousand Oaks, California: Sage Publications. Reprinted with permission of Sage Publications.

Design type	Implementation	Priority	Stage of integration	Theoretical perspective
Sequential explanatory	Quantitative followed by qualitative	Usually quantitative but can be qualitative or equal	Interpretation phase	May be present
Sequential exploratory	Qualitative followed by quantitative	Usually qualitative but can be quantitative or equal	Interpretation phase	May be present
Sequential transformative	Either qualitative followed by quantitative or quantitative followed by qualitative	Qualitative, quantitative or equal	Interpretation phase	Definitely present (i.e. conceptual framework, advocacy, empowerment)
Concurrent triangulation	Concurrent collection of quantitative and qualitative	Preferably equal, but can be quantitative or qualitative	Interpretation or analysis phase	May be present
Concurrent nested	Concurrent collection of quantitative and qualitative	Quantitative or qualitative	Analysis phase	May be present
Concurrent transformative	Concurrent collection of quantitative and qualitative	Qualitative, quantitative or equal	Usually analysis phase but can be during the interpretation phase	Definitely present (i.e. conceptual framework, advocacy, empowerment)

sequential explanatory and sequential transformative. The concurrent designs include concurrent triangulation, concurrent nested and concurrent transformative.

Sequential designs

Sequential designs usually involve multiple phases of data collection during which either a qualitative or quantitative data collection method dominates. The research purpose and the particular set of research questions determine the particular sequence in the data collection.

Sequential explanatory

This design is typically characterised by an initial quantitative phase, which is then followed by a qualitative data collection phase. The two methods are integrated during the interpretation phase. Findings from the qualitative study component are used to explain and contextualise the results from the quantitative study component (Box 3.2).

Box 3.2 Research in action

Neri and Kroll (2003) conducted a study where the two principal research aims were: 1) to identify the proportion of individuals with cerebral palsy, spinal cord injury, multiple sclerosis, or arthritis who report difficulties with accessing and/or utilising needed health care services; 2) to identify reasons for access or utilisation difficulties and the consequences that these may produce.

The quantitative component used a multistage, stratified, probability sampling approach. The survey identified a group of 'access-stressed' individuals who reported substantial problems in accessing and/or using health care services. The qualitative study component focused on this group to examine what specific barriers made access problematic and what consequences resulted from not receiving care when needed. Findings encompassed a broad range of barriers, for example, transportation, facility accessibility, provider disability competence (Scheer et al. 2002) and consequences of unmet access, for example, deterioration of physical functioning; work absenteeism; social isolation (Neri and Kroll 2003).

In our research we used qualitative research to sequentially inform quantitative findings. The study is a good example of how the quantitative study component identified a subpopulation that could be characterised as 'access stressed' (Neri and Kroll 2003). The combination of quantitative and qualitative methods in the context of one study enabled us to determine the magnitude, frequency and distribution of access and utilisation difficulties in this population as well as understand the scope and nature of barriers and consequences from the perspective of the respondents.

Sequential exploratory

This strategy typically consists of an initial phase of qualitative data collection that is followed by quantitative data collection. Findings from both data collection methods are analysed and integrated during an interpretation phase (Box 3.3).

Box 3.3 Research in action

Neri et al. (2005) conducted a study to inform the development of a survey tool that focused on physical activity and secondary conditions after spinal cord injury (SCI) (Ho et al. 2005). This study sought to: 1) understand the motivating and inhibiting factors to physical activity and exercise in people after spinal cord injury, and 2) develop, test and implement a survey tool that examines self-reported physical activity after SCI and its relationship with secondary conditions. In this study, the qualitative (exploratory) data collection preceded the quantitative study component. The focus groups specifically explored barriers and facilitators of exercise. Understanding these factors was critical to inform development of the survey tool, which included items on 'chronic and secondary conditions', 'health risk behaviours', 'hospital and health care utilisation', 'physical functioning', 'exercise activities and patterns', 'rehabilitative therapy', 'wheelchair use', 'community integration', 'self-efficacy' and 'demographics'.

The study conducted by Neri et al. (2005) highlights how the topical focus of the quantitative study component is informed by the exploratory findings from the qualitative component in conjunction with the literature sources. This approach allows for greater involvement or participation of service users and communities in refining study instruments and potentially raises the ecological validity of such tools. While most assessment instruments, whether they are used for clinical examinations, screenings or research activities, are purpose focused, they are rarely developed in collaboration or with input from the target population. Moreover, methods are often applied to other social environments than what they originally have been designed for. For example, the assessment of functional status in a clinical setting as operationalised by the functional independence measure (FIM), which has been adopted by many rehabilitation facilities in the US, may have little utility value in community settings, whereas functional status is influenced by a myriad of factors that are not captured by the instrument. Functional domains that are of subjective relevance, such as social participation, are not measured by the instrument (see also Ozer and Kroll 2002). A mixed methods approach allows design and calibration of an instrument that measures functional domains that are relevant to the target population in the most accessible and inclusive way.

Sequential transformative

Unlike the sequential exploratory or explanatory design, in sequential transformative designs there is not a predominant implementation sequence. This sequential design is guided by a particular theoretical orientation or advocacy lens (Hanson et al. 2005) and findings are integrated during the interpretation phase (Box 3.4).

Box 3.4 Research in action

Groleau et al. (2007) describe a sequential transformative design of the cultural influences on mental health problems and the advantages to the study of using this design. The study commenced with a quantitative telephone survey of the community which included the General Health Questionnaire. The quantitative phase of the study was followed by qualitative interviews which were theoretically driven. These interviews enabled the researchers to explore the cultural health experiences related to the non-use of mental health facilities by Vietnamese and West Indian participants living in an urban area of Montreal.

Concurrent designs

In concurrent mixed methods research strategies, qualitative and quantitative data are collected, as the name indicates, at the same time or in parallel.

Concurrent triangulation

This design involves a single study containing qualitative and quantitative data collection which is conducted at the same time. The purpose of this type of investigation is to validate the findings generated by each method through evidence produced by the other (Box 3.5).

Box 3.5 Research in action

In their longitudinal study of maternal and child well-being, McAuley et al. (2006) conducted semistructured in-depth interviews with mothers and collected quantitative data using several validated scales (e.g. Parenting Stress Index, Edinburgh Post-Natal Depression Scale (EPDS), Rosenberg Self-Esteem Scale) at the same home visit. The authors identified numerous family stressors in interviews, which were corroborated in the quantitative maternal stress index scales. Similarly, the objective measures (EPDS) addressing emotional well-being that indicated a high level of maternal depression were supported by findings from the interviews, in which mothers reported low energy levels, despondency and anxiety attacks. Other qualitative and quantitative measures regarding well-being, maternal perceptions of child development and social support showed similar convergent findings. The authors note that concurrent use of qualitative and quantitative measures adds to the depth and scope of findings.

Concurrent nested design

The term 'concurrent' indicates that both qualitative and quantitative data are being collected at the same time. However, in concurrent nested studies, one of the methods dominates whilst the other one is embedded, or nested, in it (Box 3.6). The research question to be answered by the embedded method may be of a secondary nature or address a very specific subtopic that is connected with the general research question.

Box 3.6 Research in action

Strasser et al. (2007) conducted a concurrent nested design to explore eating-related distress of advanced male cancer patients and their female partners. The primary method used in the study was focus groups which were attended by patients and their partners with the conduct of these groups and the analysis of the data based on grounded theory (qualitative) techniques. The secondary or nested focus of the study was the differences in patients' and their partners' assessment of the intensity and symptoms and degree of cachexia-related symptoms of eating-related disorders of patients. This secondary information was collected by a structured questionnaire which was completed at the time of the first focus group. The eating-related distress differed for patients and their partners as indicated in the qualitative findings, and this was complemented by the quantitative findings.

Concurrent transformative design

Unlike a sequential transformative design, in a concurrent transformative design both the qualitative and quantitative data are collected at the same time. The conduct of the study is informed by a theoretical perspective and data are integrated during the interpretation phase (Box 3.7).

Box 3.7 Research in action

Anastario and Schmalzbauer (2007) used a concurrent transformative mixed methods design in their cultural anthropological study of time allocation of Honduran immigrants. They used a time diary to examine gender variations among 34 Honduran immigrants in the time they spend on personal (e.g. commuting) and interpersonal responsibilities (e.g. care work, family). The study was guided by a participatory ethnographic philosophy. Observations and reported activities were quantitatively analysed for respondent-level reliability. The authors conclude that a better understanding of gender differences in time allocation for responsibilities will be critical to inform knowledge about health outcome disparities.

Some additional designs

There are additional research designs such as ethnography, case study, evaluation studies and action research that may use qualitative and quantitative methods in the one study. Moreover, some research identified as using case study, evaluation or action research, could also be categorised into one of the six designs identified as common to mixed methods research. Additionally, case study and evaluation studies may not be linked to a specific paradigm and therefore could be encompassed under a pragmatic paradigm. Rosenberg and Yates (2007), for example, view case study as a method (and not a methodology) that is 'pragmatically – rather than paradigmatically – driven' (p. 448), which clearly places this design as underpinned by pragmatism and therefore under the mixed methods research umbrella. As a number of case studies is undertaken for the purpose of evaluation this may apply to evaluation studies. Similarly, action research and ethnographic studies that utilise mixed methods in their data collection may be aligned to mixed methods research. More debate is required about the positioning of the many other types of designs that integrate qualitative and quantitative methods in their research design.

Data collection methods

Designs are often equated with methods. However, it is important to distinguish clearly between the features of the research design and the methods that populate a design with data. Both design and method are linked to the research purpose, and more specifically to the research question. Generally, multiple methods of data collection can find application within a particular design. Interviews, observational methods, document analyses, physiological measures can be used in the context of experimental, longitudinal, case control or cross-sectional designs. However, the research question determines *how* they are used and in *what way* the data generated by these methods will provide answers.

As has been demonstrated throughout this chapter, it is important that the choice of method(s) is appropriate to address the specific study questions. In fact, the research objective, research questions, design and choice of method need to follow a consistent rationale, and data collection and analysis need to be realistic and feasible considering time and resources available.

Future developments

Mixed methods designs clearly have significant potential to facilitate the development of knowledge in nursing and the health sciences. However, while currently mixed methods designs are understood as a combination of qualitative and quantitative methods it may well be extended to other methodological combinations within one particular study. Equally thinkable are QUAN–QUAN–QUAL studies or QUAL–QUAL–QUAN studies (Box 3.8).

For example, a rehabilitation researcher may struggle with an underpowered randomised controlled study that produced no significant differences between an intervention and a control group. However, upon examination the researcher may find that some of the cases in the intervention group are interesting 'outliers'. These may be followed up longitudinally within a single subject case study producing additional quantitative data and in-depth qualitative interviews to explore the mechanisms underlying their behaviour even further. Similarly, a meta-synthesis may provide a good understanding of a phenomenon based on the interpretation of qualitative research findings from multiple studies, which in turn may be followed an in-depth qualitative exploration of additional topics. Findings from the primary data collection effort may strengthen interpretations of the original meta-synthesis and may then lead to the formulation of quantitative survey items.

Box 3.8 Research in action

Gulmans et al. (2007) discuss the potential for a multiphase evaluation study of patient care communication in integrated care settings using a sequential three-step mixed design (QUAN–QUAL–QUAL). Integrated care settings typically involve multiple professions and multidirectional communication links with which the patient has to interact. Patients hold specific expectations with regard to care settings. A quality gap arises when these expectations are not met, and the experiences differ. Care pathways and the number of communication links between patient and health professionals differ in complexity for various conditions (e.g. stroke, diabetes). In a first step, the authors suggest conducting a quality evaluation of communication from the perspective of the service user using a tailored questionnaire to identify potential quality gaps (QUAN). In-depth interviews (QUAL) with a subset of patients will then be used to illuminate the mechanisms that may be responsible for the mismatch between expectancies and experiences. The final evaluation step involves focus groups with health care professionals (QUAL) to examine findings from the previous two steps, to add the professional viewpoint and to identify solutions to close the quality gap.

Conclusion

It is evident that many current national health research priorities favour mixed methods designs. The UK's Medical Research Council's Framework for the Design and Evaluation of Complex Health Interventions (Campbell et al. 2007) builds on a phased approach. In the pre-experimental stages there is sufficient scope for exploratory work that draws on mixed methods and at the trial stage, qualitative study components may complement findings from the clinical experimental testing. The application of mixed methods designs as part of multiyear research and development projects, described earlier, may be reflective of such a phased approach (Nastasi et al. 2007).

In the scientific literature there has been a steady increase in the volume of mixed methods research published over the past decade and this trend is likely to continue. The field will probably continue to mature in terms of designs and integration practice. Mixed methods designs are also increasingly taught as part of curricula in research methods courses. The growing popularity of mixed methods research is reflected in the increasing number of higher degree research theses that employ these methods. Care needs to be taken, however, to ensure that scholarly discourse is undertaken to facilitate the development of rigorous methodological frameworks to support the creativity of mixed methods research.

References

Anastario M. and Schmalzbauer L. (2007) Piloting the time diary method among Honduran immigrants: gendered time use. *Journal of Immigrant and Minority Health*. Accessed 1 April 2007 at www.springerlink.com/content/21717hn4n7444780.

Andrew S. and Halcomb E.J. (2007) Mixed methods research is an effective method of enquiry for community health nursing. *Contemporary Nurse*, **23**, 145–153.

Bandura A. (1997) *Self-Efficacy: The Exercise of Control*. New York: W.H. Freeman.

Campbell N., Murray E., Darbyshire J. et al. (2007) Designing and evaluating complex interventions to improve health care. *British Medical Journal*, **334**, 455–459.

Creswell J.W. (2003) *Research Design: Qualitative, Quantitative and Mixed Methods Approaches*. Thousand Oaks, California: Sage Publications.

Creswell J.W., Plano Clark V.L., Gutmann M.L. and Hanson W.E. (2003) Advanced mixed methods research designs. In Tashakkori A. and Teddlie C. (eds.) *Handbook of Mixed Methods in Social and Behavioral Research*, pp. 209–240. Thousand Oaks, California: Sage Publications.

Groleau D., Pluye P. and Nadueau L. (2007) A mix-method approach to the cultural understanding of distress and the non-use of mental health services. *Journal of Mental Health*, **16**(6), 731–741.

Gulmans J., Vollenbroek-Hutten M.M.R., Van Gemert-Pijnen J.E.W.C. and Van Harten W.H. (2007) Evaluating quality of patient care communication in integrated care settings: a mixed method approach. *International Journal for Quality in Health Care*, **19**(5), 281–288.

Hakim C. (1987) *Research Design. Strategies and Choices in the Design of Social Research*. London: Allan and Unwin.

Hanson W.E., Creswell J.W., Plano Clark V.L., Petska K.S. and Creswell J.D. (2005) Mixed methods research designs in counseling psychology. *Journal of Counseling Psychology*, **52**(2), 224–235.

Ho P.-S., Neri M., Kroll T. and Kehn M. (2005) *Enhancing content validity and relevance of surveys through consumer participation: Development of a survey for people with spinal cord injury*. Paper presented at the American Public Health Association's 133rd Annual Meeting, Philadelphia, PA.

Kroll T., Neri M.T. and Miller K. (2005) Using mixed methods in disability and rehabilitation research. *Rehabilitation Nursing*, **30**(3), 106–113.

McAuley C., McCurry N., Knapp M., Beecham J. and Sleed M. (2006) Young families under stress: assessing maternal and child well-being using a mixed-methods approach. *Child and Family Social Work*, **11**, 43–54.

Minkler M. and Wallerstein N. (2003) Introduction to community based participatory research. In Minkler M. and Wallerstein N. (eds.) *Community-Based Participatory Research for Health*, pp. 3–26. San Francisco: Jossey-Bass.

Nastasi B.K., Hitchcock J., Sreeroopa S., Burkholder G., Varjas K. and Jayasena A. (2007) Mixed methods in intervention research: theory to adaptation. *Journal of Mixed Methods Research*, **1**(2), 164–182.

Neri M.T. and Kroll T. (2003) Understanding the consequences of access barriers to health care: experiences of adults with disabilities. *Disability and Rehabilitation*, **25**(2), 85–96.

Neri M.T., Kroll T. and Groah S. (2005) Towards consumer-defined exercise programs for people with spinal cord injury: focus group findings. *Journal of Spinal Cord Medicine*, **28**(2), 132.

Newman I., Ridenour C.S., Newman C. and DeMarco jr. G.M. (2003) A typology of research purposes and its relationship to mixed methods. In Tashakkori A. and Teddlie C. (eds.) *Handbook of Mixed Methods in Social and Behavioral Research*, pp. 167–188. Thousand Oaks, California: Sage.

Ozer M. and Kroll T. (2002) Patient-centered rehabilitation: problems and opportunities. *Critical Reviews in Physical and Rehabilitation Medicine*, **14**(3–4), 221–230.

Priestley M. (2003) *Disability: A Life Course Approach*. Cambridge, UK: Polity.

Rosenberg J.P. and Yates P.M. (2007) Schematic representation of case study research designs. *Journal of Advanced Nursing*, **60**(4), 447–452.

Robson C. (2002) *Real World Research: A Resource Guide for Social Scientists and Practitioner Researchers*, 2nd edition. Oxford: Blackwell Science.

Scheer J., Kroll T., Neri M. and Beatty P. (2002) Access barriers for persons with disabilities: the consumer perspective. *Journal of Disability Policy Studies*, **13**(4), 221–230.

Schensul S.L., Nastasi B.K. and Verma R.K. (2006) Community-based research in India, a case example of international and transdisciplinary collaboration. *American Journal of Community Psychology*, **38**, 95–111.

Strasser F., Binswanger J. and Cerny T. (2007) Fighting a losing battle: eating-related distress of men with advances cancer and their female partners. A mixed-methods study. *Palliative Medicine*, **21**, 129–137.

Tashakkori A. and Teddlie C. (eds.) (2003) *Handbook of Mixed Methods in Social and Behavioral Research*, pp. 167–188. Thousand Oaks, California: Sage.

Managing Mixed Methods Projects

Elizabeth J. Halcomb and Sharon Andrew

Learning objectives

After reading this chapter, you will have the knowledge to:

a) State the key considerations in identifying a research problem.
b) Describe the use of literature in the development of a research proposal.
c) Identify the steps in reviewing the literature.
d) Describe the structure of a mixed methods research proposal.
e) Identify considerations in presenting a mixed methods research proposal.
f) Describe the human and physical resource considerations of mixed methods research.
g) Discuss the role of research teams in mixed methods research.
h) Understand the ethical considerations related to mixed methods designs.

Introduction

Mixed methods research requires meticulous planning if a project is to be conducted successfully. Beyond the general requirements of research, in terms of having a realistic problem of sufficient interest and the ability and resources to gather the required information, consideration needs to be given to the management of the extensive data collected during the course of a mixed methods investigation. Mixed methods research is likely to be more costly to conduct in terms of the time, skills and resources required compared to a purely qualitative or quantitative study. However, this should be outweighed by the greater insight into the research problem than would have been achieved with a purely quantitative or qualitative investigation. This chapter will explore some of the pragmatic research management issues that researchers may face when conducting mixed methods research and provide guidance in addressing these issues throughout the research process.

The mixed methods research proposal

A research proposal is a document that supports the need to conduct a study and describes and justifies the proposed research process. The proposal identifies the research problem and provides a synthesis of the relevant literature, as well as providing justification of the proposed methodology, a description of proposed data collection methods, a projected budget and timeline and identification of potential outcomes from the research. The research proposal is developed before the study commences, usually as part of an application for approval to conduct the study from a Human Research Ethics Committee. Some higher education institutions require their postgraduate students to submit a written proposal and/or present their proposal orally before confirming their candidature and undertaking the research. Here we examine the nature of a mixed methods research proposal which, while similar to purely qualitative or quantitative studies, has some specific considerations.

Proposal structure

The structure of a mixed methods proposal may differ from that of a single method study. The proposal may be influenced by the research design including the sequence of the data collection, the priority assigned to the data and how and where the data are integrated. We suggest that the researcher develops a framework akin to a 'road map' for the proposal. This may assist the reader or those required to assess the proposal by giving a visual depiction of how and when the different aspects of data collection will occur, including any variations in the study samples, timing, priority and study locations. As there are often word or page limits on a research proposal, a visual depiction can assist in providing a succinct summary of the material being discussed.

The research problem

The increasing age of the population and rise in chronic and complex disease states has led researchers to recognise that a growing number of health-related research problems require multiple approaches. These reasons, combined with those presented in Chapter 1 (namely increased reflexivity in relationships; increased political awareness; growing formalisation of research governance; new technologies; governance; and international research collaboration) have resulted in an increased interest in mixed methods research.

In mixed methods, like all research, the fundamental driver for choosing a particular research design is the nature of the research problem. The research problem must merit a mixed methods approach and a researcher must consider whether this approach will add a unique dimension to findings that a quantitative or qualitative design alone will not sufficiently provide. Creswell and Plano Clark (2006) assert that a research problem requires a mixed methods approach when: 1) the research problem requires a combination of qualitative and quantitative data to provide an adequate answer; 2) a secondary form of data is needed within a design; 3) quantitative results need to be explained with qualitative data; or 4) an initial qualitative investigation is required to inform the development of a quantitative study.

It is not justifiable to choose a mixed methods approach to simply add padding to a thesis or to 'prop up' a weak study which has methodological flaws. The researcher must be able to substantiate why a mixed methods design is necessary and articulate what this design adds to the explanation or understanding of the research problem.

Reasons for using a mixed methods design

There are six primary purposes generally proposed in the literature for using mixed methods designs: 1) confirmation, 2) complementarity, 3) initiation, 4) development, 5) expansion (Greene et al. 1989), and 6) enhancement of significant findings (Onwuegbuzie and Leech 2004). We propose that the sixth reason be modified to enhancement of significant or non-significant findings (Andrew et al. 2007). Mixed methods research is not limited to a single purpose for conducting a study as there may be multiple reasons for using this methodology (Andrew and Halcomb 2006, 2007). Table 4.1 presents some common rationales for conducting mixed methods research.

Confirmation

In a mixed methods study conducted for the purpose of confirmation, the focus of the qualitative and quantitative data is on the same phenomena. The findings from the different data collection methods are expected to converge, thereby confirming and increasing the validity of the findings (Denzin 1989).

Complementarity

If one method will only explain an aspect of a problem then complementary data may be collected to elaborate, enhance or clarify the findings from the primary method (Greene and Caracelli 1989; Morgan 1998). This rationale is commonly used in studies where the dominant data collection method is quantitative and qualitative data are used to explain or expand the quantitative findings.

Initiation

Qualitative and quantitative data may be required to explore a research problem as there may be areas where little is known about the problem, or about one dimension of the problem only. Rather than looking for consistency in findings, studies for the purpose of initiation seek to find contradiction, inconsistencies or a new perspective to a research problem (Greene et al. 1989; Onwuegbuzie and Leech 2004).

Development

Mixed methods studies may be used for the purpose of the development of a research instrument. Qualitative data may be collected to explore the research problem through the identification of key concepts that will then assist in the formation of quantitative instrument items.

Expansion

Qualitative and quantitative methods focus on different areas of the research problem with the purpose of broadening the scope of the

Table 4.1 Reasons for conducting mixed methods studies. Adapted from: Andrew and Halcomb 2006; Creswell and Plano Clark 2006.

Research problem	Purpose	Example
Qualitative or quantitative data alone will not fully explain the research problem	Complementarity	This design is commonly used in quantitative dominant studies with qualitative data used to explain or expand the quantitative findings. Halcomb et al. (2008b) conducted a national survey of Australian practice nurses to describe their demographic and employment characteristics and their role in clinical practice. Telephone interviews were conducted after the survey to further explore the nurses' role and the barriers and facilitators to role development (Halcomb et al. 2008a)
Qualitative and quantitative data are required to explore the research problem with a greater depth and breadth	Initiation	To study the burden of percutaneous endoscopic gastrostomies from a patient perspective, Jordan et al. (2006) used a combination of validated tools and interviews. The addition of quantitative data in this study identified some significant and treatable problems not mentioned by participants in the interviews
Developing a research instrument	Development	In her study of nurses' perceptions of quality and the factors that affect quality of care for older people living in long-term care settings in Ireland, Murphy (2007) developed her quantitative questionnaire from data that had been previously generated via interviews
Qualitative and quantitative methods focus on different areas of the research problem	Expansion	To explore depression amongst veterans recovering from stroke Williams et al. (2005) combined quantitative data from the geriatric depression scale and medical record audit with qualitative interview data to gain a more detailed understanding of depression during stroke recovery
The focus is on the same phenomena with data collected by both qualitative and quantitative methods	Confirmation	Hatonen et al. (2008) used a combination of structured and open-ended questions to explore the experiences of patient education during inpatient mental health care
Additional data are required to enhance understanding of the primary data findings	Enhance significant findings	A study includes a secondary method of data collection to explain or explore the primary data findings. For example, a randomised controlled trial may incorporate qualitative data to explain non-compliance in the study protocol

study (Greene et al. 1989). Integration occurs in separate findings or a discussion chapter.

Enhancement of significant findings

A mixed methods study may be undertaken with the purpose of enhancing significant statistical, practical, clinical or economical findings. Onwuegbuzie and Leech (2004) suggest that a intervention study, for example, may have non-significant statistical findings but the intervention may have clinical significance and a mixed methods study may assist in understanding the study results. Moreover, a mixed methods study may be conducted with the purpose of identifying and exploring the 'statistically non-significant' or 'extreme' cases.

Problem statement

The introduction to the research proposal introduces the reader to the research problem. The general structure of the introduction is a transition from a description of the broad nature of the problem to a more specific statement about the problem (problem statement). The beginning sentences, for example, may include statistics to support the importance of the problem nationally and/or worldwide or about the historical importance of the topic of interest. This may be followed by paragraphs introducing key concepts and variables and then focus on the key elements specific to the study problem. Throughout this discussion the need for the study and any gaps in the literature or knowledge that are evident are subtly introduced and reinforced. The introduction should conclude with a paragraph summarising the key elements of the problem that are specific to the study and a statement about how the study will address this problem (purpose statement). The problem statement should provide some justification for the consideration of a mixed methods design for the investigation of the problem.

Purpose statement

The purpose statement is concerned with the aim or intent of the study. This statement may be found in the concluding sentences of the introduction, as a separate subsection (labelled purpose or aim of the study), or at the beginning of the method section of the research proposal. The purpose statement generally identifies the phenomena or variables being studied, the population and setting. A mixed methods study should have an overarching statement that encompasses the primary purpose of the study (Box 4.1). Following this, separate statements may describe the qualitative and quantitative sections of the project. It is useful to articulate clearly how these statements link to the subsequent data collection to avoid any confusion by the reader about the course of the project.

Box 4.1 Research in action

In a mixed methods study of the development of expertise in heart failure self-care, Riegel et al. (2007) include their detailed research purpose statement in the methods section of their manuscript. The statement begins with an overarching statement: 'Using a mixed-methods (qualitative and quantitative) design . . . the decision-making processes used by patients were explored' (p. 136). The authors then elaborate the aims of the quantitative and qualitative data collection aspects of the study.

Research questions

We believe in addition to an overarching study purpose, a mixed methods study should also have a single overarching research question, which describes the research problem that the entire study is setting out to address. This question should guide the researcher in the primary reasons for the study. The researcher should be pragmatic in how the question is framed, that is, where possible it should support the mixing of paradigms in preference to giving the appearance of preferring one particular paradigm. The study may have additional subquestions that specifically drive the different methods of data collection utilised in the study. That is, there may be questions for the qualitative and quantitative aspects of the study, and each must be congruent with their concomitant paradigm. The quantitative aspect of the study may also have hypotheses.

Literature and the development of a research proposal

The peer-reviewed literature is essential for developing two distinct aspects of research proposal development, namely: 1) defining the scope of the research problem; and 2) supporting the choice of research design and data collection methods.

A critical literature review relating to the research problem should be undertaken as would be done for purely qualitative or quantitative research to synthesise current knowledge and identify the gap that the proposed study seeks to address (Carnwell and Daly 2001). However, consideration should be given to identifying and contrasting qualitative and quantitative findings to provide justification for the selection of a mixed methods design.

Given the relatively new nature of mixed methods research in many disciplines, it is important that researchers learn from each other and contribute to scholarly discourse related to the design, implementation and presentation of mixed methods research. The peer-reviewed literature is an important reference source on issues pertaining to methodology as well as research problems.

Steps in reviewing the literature

Searching for the literature

Increasingly, literature reviews undertaken in the development of a research proposal are expected to be methodical in their approach, with a clearly defined and justified scope and limitations. The reader needs to be convinced that the research team have thoroughly explored the body of literature in order to define the context of their study (Steward 2004). This can be achieved by providing details and justification of the search strategy used, including search terms, inclusion/exclusion criteria, limits of search (e.g. dates of publication, languages) and databases examined (Steward 2004). In mixed methods research this kind of definition may be particularly important considering the complexity of research problems being addressed or multiple perspectives being considered within a single study. Also, mixed methods research may rely on a range of sources, including less conventional 'literature' such as letters, documents, newspaper reports and art works to set the scene for the work that may need to be included in the review (Mauch and Birch 1998).

Whilst it is not necessary for literature reviews in mixed methods studies to focus only on other mixed methods investigations, the critical review of mixed methods studies may be relevant in assisting in the development of the research method or addressing practical issues. Identification of mixed methods studies in many electronic databases is not as straightforward as one might imagine, and so is worthy of some consideration here. This difficulty is the result of the diverse terminology used to describe mixed methods research in the electronic databases, the publication bias that often leads to papers reporting

Table 4.2 Search strategies for identifying mixed methods research.

Search term	Rationale
mixed method*	* acts as a wildcard and retrieves terms including 'mixed method', 'mixed methodology' and 'mixed methods research'
quantitative AND qualitative	AND acts as a Boolean operator and retrieves all citations that have a keyword of quantitative and a keyword of qualitative. If this reveals too many citations other combinations of common mixed methods data collection techniques (e.g. interviews and surveys) can be used to narrow the search
multimethod	Although multimethod may be used as a keyword to identify citations in some electronic databases the true meaning of multimethod research includes those studies that collect data using two or more data collection methods from the same research tradition (e.g. interviews and participant observation)

separate rather than mixed datasets and the 'new' nature of the mixed methods research. Additionally, it is not uncommon for qualitative and quantitative findings, of what would otherwise be considered a mixed methods study, to be reported in separate papers (Clendon 2004; Clendon and Krothe 2004; Krothe and Clendon 2006; Polit and Beck 2006). Table 4.2 provides some suggested search terms that could be used to identify mixed methods research within electronic databases. Whilst such terms provide some general guidance, they would need to be considered in relation to the specific nomenclature used in the database being searched.

Appraising mixed methods literature

A preliminary appraisal of the literature would include identification that qualitative and quantitative data have been used in the reported study. This may appear elementary but from our experience there is still some confusion and variability in the use of the term mixed methods. Chapters 7 and 8 contain material that will assist a researcher to appraise mixed methods studies reported in the literature.

Ethical considerations related to mixed methods designs

Whilst the ethical issues encountered in mixed methods investigations are essentially the same as those confronting the researcher conducting purely qualitative or quantitative investigations, there are some additional issues that require consideration.

The proposal seeking approval from a Human Research Ethics Committee to conduct a mixed methods study may be complex as there will be two methods of data collection to be discussed, including the recruitment of study participants, comments about the sample size, data collection instruments and data analysis. The researcher must decide whether to combine the data collection procedures on the one application or to submit separate applications for the separate arms of the study. This decision will depend upon the exact nature of the study. For example, if both sets of data are to be collected from the same individuals at the same time then it would be advisable to submit one application. On the other hand if the data collection is to be conducted sequentially and there may be a time lag in this process then it may be more expedient to submit separate proposals for each study arm. If one application is made for both the qualitative and quantitative data collection the researcher may be required to clearly articulate the connection between the study arms.

The researcher must justify the value a mixed methods approach will have in answering the research question. The need to use both quantitative and qualitative data must be clear, particularly in terms of the potentially increased burden to participants from collecting two datasets. Any ambiguities noted by an ethics committee may be similar to those which a manuscript reviewer or dissertation examiner may identify.

Health research participants may have a range of co-morbidities or social issues that must be considered in any data collection procedure. Where participants are being requested to participate in both the qualitative and quantitative aspects of a mixed methods study, the burden of this participation must be considered. Ethics committees may want assurance that the researcher has considered this and taken steps to minimise the burden.

Where participants for the second data collection are generated from within those who participate in the initial data collection, strategies need to be implemented to capture contact details from participants separate to their study data. Local legislation and Ethics Committee preferences can guide how this can be achieved without compromising participants' privacy and confidentiality.

Human and physical resource considerations of mixed methods research

Researcher skills

The conduct of a mixed methods study requires the researcher to be competent in both qualitative and quantitative research methods. If an individual researcher does not have these skills then there is a need to acquire them, seek mentorship from a supervision team with such skills or consider convening a team of researchers with complementary skills to support the conduct of the study. Postgraduate higher degree research candidates must seriously consider their current skills and establish a clear plan for skill development if they are considering undertaking mixed methods research. Important skills are not limited to data collection or analysis techniques but also include an understanding of the paradigm issues and how they will influence congruence in the study and skills to facilitate true integration and mixing of methods.

Postgraduate research students planning to undertake a mixed methods study should also consider the methodological expertise of their supervisory team. Students should seek not only academics who have high level qualitative or quantitative skills, but at least one supervisor who has an interest and experience in mixed methods research. Consideration of the compatibility of potential supervisors with both your research topic area and each others' worldview and methodological expertise is important if you are to have a productive candidature.

Time

Researchers must consider the time involved in the conduct of a mixed methods study. The collection of data through different procedures will logically require more time than a single method study (Connelly et al. 1997). The use of a sequential design will also be more time consuming, as datasets are collected one after the other. Therefore, during the planning phase, it is essential that a timeline be developed to map out the anticipated progress of the study. This is particularly important to ensure that reporting deadlines for funding bodies and milestones related to research candidatures can be achieved.

The development of a timeline before the commencement of the research will also enable the researcher to consider where time can be saved during the course of the study. For example, a researcher may be able to combine recruitment of participant samples to be used in the study or data entry can be undertaken whilst the literature review is being written into a paper for publication. This can be important to ensure that the research is conducted efficiently and within time limitations.

Financial considerations

A combination of data collection methods may increase significantly the costs associated with a mixed methods study (Duffy 1987; Redfern and Norman 1994). However, some funding bodies are increasingly giving preference to mixed methods investigations. The preparation of a budget during the planning phase will give the researcher a detailed understanding of the costs predicted to be incurred during the study. It can also highlight areas where costs might be able to be reduced, or where additional funding could be sought to reduce burden on the researcher (e.g. data entry).

Research teams

As is the case in any research, the quality of the proposal or study will, at least in part, be judged by the track record and credibility of the researchers. Few researchers have expertise in both qualitative and quantitative methods, therefore, for the most part, collaboration will be required to conduct mixed methods research effectively (Todd et al. 2004). Given the complexity, unique skills and specific considerations related to integration and true mixing of qualitative and quantitative data it would be optimal if at least one member of this team has skills in mixed methods research. The increasing popularity of mixed methods will assist in developing the skills of those with an interest in mixed methods, thus increasing the number of researchers with such methodological expertise. It is our observation, however, that the quality of different researchers' experience in mixed methods research is variable. Care should be taken to evaluate the quality of individual researchers' experiences before engaging their expertise in the area.

Building a strong team with the requisite methodological and clinical expertise is likely to bring together several researchers, each with different strengths and skills (Twinn 2003). These researchers may come from different disciplines, and may be situated in different locations. It is important that they have the desire to work together to achieve a common goal and have the ability to work within the philosophical underpinnings of mixed methods research. For some, who have strong beliefs and paradigmatic allegiances, this might be extremely difficult. If not appropriately managed, such conflict can create serious divisions within the research team and can even thwart the success of the entire project. Any discipline or work cultures must also be addressed for a team to work productively.

Teams engaged in mixed methods research must work collaboratively to ensure that the research plan is clearly conceptualised and the study design is defined and justified. It is essential that an effective team leader is identified to facilitate the conduct of the study. In addition to developing a coherent research plan, the research team must decide how they will implement this plan. These decisions will be driven by the research question and study design but may also be influenced by factors such as the composition of the team, the locations of various team members, access to participant groups and other workload commitments. For example, different members may conduct various data collections and analyses based on their individual methodological expertise or team members located in two cities may collect identical datasets from their two locations to facilitate comparison between the two groups. Regardless of how the workload for the project is divided, the team leader must ensure that all members contribute to the project in a way that is acceptable to the team. The team must also meet regularly to share thoughts, ideas and plan the integration of study findings.

As in any research where there are multiple researchers, authorship for any papers arising from the study must be established early to prevent any conflicts or disagreements. Guidelines such as the *Uniform Requirements for Manuscripts Submitted to Biomedical Journals: Writing and Editing for Biomedical Publication* should be used to direct decisions regarding individual contributions and authorship (International Committee of Medical Journal Editors 2007). A more detailed discussion regarding publication of mixed methods findings can be found in Chapter 8.

Conclusion

This chapter has presented some of the practical considerations that need to be explored during the planning of a mixed methods project. Giving adequate thought to these factors during the planning and development phases can significantly reduce problems encountered during the conduct of the study. The time and effort needed to explore these factors and plan for a mixed methods investigation should not be underestimated, but neither should the value of this to the conduct of the study.

References

Andrew S. and Halcomb E.J. (2006) Mixed methods research is an effective method of enquiry for working with families and communities. *Contemporary Nurse*, **23**, 145–153.

Andrew S. and Halcomb E.J. (2007) Mixed method research. In Borbasi S. and Jackson D. (eds.) *Navigating the Maze of Nursing Research: An Interactive Learning Adventure*, 2nd edition, pp. 178–200. Marrickville, New South Wales: Elsevier.

Andrew S., Salamonson Y. and Halcomb E.J. (2008) Nursing students' maths self-efficacy: Psychometric testing of the NSE-Maths instrument. *Nurse Education Today*. In press.

Carnwell R. and Daly W.M. (2001) Strategies for the construction of a critical review of the literature. *Nurse Education in Practice*, **2**, 57–63.

Clendon J. (2004) Demonstrating outcomes in a nurse-led clinic: how primary health care nurses make a difference to children and their families. *Contemporary Nurse*, **18**, 164–176.

Clendon J. and Krothe J. (2004) The nurse-managed clinic: an evaluative study. *Nursing Praxis in New Zealand*, **20**, 15–23.

Connelly L.M., Bott M., Hoffart N. and Taunton R.L. (1997) Methodological triangulation in a study of nurse retention. *Nursing Research*, **46**, 299–302.

Creswell J.W. and Plano Clark V. (2006) *Designing and Conducting Mixed Methods Research*. Thousand Oaks, California: Sage Publications.

Denzin N.K. (1989) *The Research Act: A Theoretical Introduction to Sociological Methods*. Englewood Cliffs, New Jersey: Prentice Hall.

Duffy M.E. (1987) Methodological triangulation: a vehicle for merging quantitative and qualitative research methods. *IMAGE: Journal of Nursing Scholarship*, **9**, 130–133.

Greene J.C. and Caracelli V.J. (eds.) (1989) *Advances in Mixed Methods Evaluation: The Challenges and Benefits of Integrating Diverse Paradigms*. San Francisco: Jossey-Bass.

Greene J.C., Caracelli V.J. and Graham W.F. (1989) Toward a conceptual framework for mixed-method evaluation designs. *Educational Evaluation and Policy Analysis*, **11**, 255–274.

Halcomb E.J., Davidson P.M., Griffiths R. and Daly J. (2008a) Cardiovascular disease management: time to advance the practice nurse role? *Australian Health Review*, **32**, 44–55.

Halcomb E.J., Davidson P.M., Salamonson Y. and Ollerton R. (2008b) Nurses in Australian general practice: implications for chronic disease management. *Journal of Nursing and Healthcare of Chronic Illness*, in association with *Journal of Clinical Nursing*, **17**, 6–15.

Hatonen H., Kuosmanen L., Malkavaara H. and Valimaki M. (2008) Mental health: patients' experiences of patient education during inpatient care. *Journal of Clinical Nursing*, **17**, 752–762.

International Committee of Medical Journal Editors (2007) *Uniform Requirements for Manuscripts Submitted to Biomedical Journals: Writing and Editing for Biomedical Publication*. http://www.icmje.org/.

Jordan S., Philpin S., Warring J., Cheung W.Y. and Williams J.M.A. (2006) Percutaneous endoscopic gastrostomies: the burden of treatment from a patient perspective. *Journal of Advanced Nursing*, **56**, 270–281.

Krothe J.S. and Clendon J. (2006) Perceptions of effectiveness of nurse-managed clinics: a cross-cultural study. *Public Health Nursing*, **23**, 242–249.

Mauch J.E. and Birch J.W. (1998) *Guide to the Successful Thesis and Dissertation: A Handbook for Students and Faculty*. New York: Marcel Dekker, Inc.

Morgan D.L. (1998) Practical strategies for combining qualitative and quantitative methods: applications to health research. *Qualitative Health Research*, **8**, 362–376.

Murphy K. (2007) Nurses' perceptions of quality and the factors that affect quality care for older people living in long-term care settings in Ireland. *Journal of Clinical Nursing*, **16**, 873–884.

Onwuegbuzie A.J. and Leech N.L. (2004) Enhancing the interpretation of 'significant' findings: the role of mixed methods research. *The Qualitative Report*, **9**, 770–792.

Polit D.F. and Beck C.T. (2006) *Essentials of Nursing Research: Methods, Appraisal and Utilization*. Philadelphia: Lippincott Williams and Wilkins.

Redfern S.J. and Norman I.J. (1994) Validity through triangulation. *Nurse Researcher*, **2**, 41–56.

Riegel B., Dickson V.V., Goldberg L.R. and Deatrick J.A. (2007) Factors associated with the development of expertise in health failure self-care. *Nursing Research*, **56**, 235–243.

Steward B. (2004) Writing a literature review. *British Journal of Occupational Therapy*, **67**, 495–500.

Todd Z., Nerlich B., McKeown S. and Clarke D.D. (2004) *Mixing Methods in Psychology: The Integration of Qualitative and Quantitative Methods in Theory and Practice*. New York: Taylor and Francis Group.

Twinn S. (2003) Status of mixed methods in research in nursing. In Tashakkori A. and Teddlie C. (eds.) *Handbook of Mixed Methods in Social and Behavioral Research*, pp. 541–556. California: Sage Books.

Williams C.L., Rittman M.R., Boylstein C., Faircloth C. and Haijing Q. (2005) Qualitative and quantitative measurement of depression in veterans recovering from stroke. *Journal of Rehabilitation Research and Development*, **42**, 277–290.

Section Two

Conducting Mixed Methods Research

Data Collection in Mixed Methods Research

Julia Brannen and Elizabeth J. Halcomb

Learning objectives

The aim of this chapter is to provide the reader with a practical understanding of data collection methods applied to mixed methods investigations. After reading this chapter, you will have the knowledge to:

a) Identify some ways of collecting data in mixed methods research.
b) Clarify the purposes of each data collection method in relation to a mixed method research design.
c) Understand how a mixed method design influences decisions concerning data collection.
d) Discuss the concept of sampling in mixed methods research.
e) Appreciate the need for reflectivity and a careful consideration of ethical issues in mixed methods research.

Introduction

In addition to the decisions around study design, the mixed methods researcher must also select and implement methods to collect the qualitative and quantitative data for their study. This chapter will explore how the use of a mixed methods design impacts upon the collection of study data. It will discuss some of the fundamental issues faced by researchers collecting both qualitative and quantitative data in a mixed methods study and identify some strategies to address these issues.

Considerations for data collection

The underlying premise behind using a mixed methods design is that it allows the researcher to collect data that will best answer the research question (Brannen 2004, Brannen 2005, McEvoy and Richards 2006). To this end, the qualitative and quantitative data collection must, in some way, provide a more complete picture of the research problem than would have been possible through the collection of either type of data alone. As has been discussed in Chapter 3, the nature of the research question and the reasons for choosing a mixed methods approach both impact on the choice of study design. Whilst the study design provides a framework for the sequencing of data collection, relative priority of datasets and the stages of integration, careful planning of mixed data collection is required. Such planning must consider the range of theoretical and practical considerations discussed below.

Data collection methods

Implicit in mixed methods research is the concept that both qualitative and quantitative data will be collected. In choosing data collection methods there is an opportunity for the researcher to be creative in their approach and combination of specific techniques. Common methods to collect quantitative data include standardised scales, checklists/inventories, self-reports/surveys or rating scales. Qualitative data can be collected via interview, open-ended written questions, focus groups, journals/diaries, observation, meeting transcripts, literature or art works. Increasingly, technology is promoting innovation in some of these traditional methods of data collection with a growing number of studies collecting data via email, blogs and other forms of electronic communication (for example, Constantino et al. 2007; Drummond et al. 2007). Such innovation is certainly an excellent opportunity for researchers to collect data from hard-to-reach groups and employ creativity in methods of collecting data. Regardless of the method chosen, each has a number of advantages and limitations as can be seen in Table 5.1.

In many instances the collection of mixed data will be achieved through the use of two or more complementary methods of data collection that separately collect qualitative and quantitative data either sequentially or concurrently (e.g. interviews and validated instrument,

Table 5.1 Advantages and disadvantages of data collection methods.

Data collection method	Advantages	Disadvantages
Interviews	Response rate relatively higher Clarification of responses can be undertaken	Potential for interviewer bias Relatively expensive to undertake
Focus groups	Group discussion can yield different information from individual interviews Large number of informants can participate in a short period of time	Participants may disagree with the consensus and remain silent Individual participants may take over the discussion
Questionnaires/surveys	Relatively cheap to administer Offer complete anonymity No interviewer bias as often self-administered Can reach a wider population than face-to-face data collection	Response rate can be relatively lower than face-to-face data collection Clarification of responses or non-response to certain items cannot be sought Forces respondent to choose from pre-determined responses
Validated tests/scales	Instrument validity and reliability established Can provide data that can be compared against established norms	Temptation to try and 'fit' research question to available instruments Scale norms may not 'fit' the groups studied
Observation	Participants observed during their daily interactions Potential to provide depth and variety of information about area of interest	Potential for observer bias Relatively expensive to undertake Likely to be very time consuming Ethical considerations

focus groups and survey tools). This model of data collection generally involves using separate data collection strategies that collect purely qualitative or quantitative data (Johnson and Turner 2003). Additionally, multiple methods of data collection can be used to generate several datasets. Such data collection has obvious implications for resources, duration of projects and the need for dual sampling. An alternative strategy that could be considered is the collection of some, or all, of the qualitative and quantitative data during the same data collection encounter (see example in Brannen 2004). As can be seen in

Table 5.2, many data collection strategies that are commonly associated with either the positivist or naturalistic paradigm, can be adapted to collect data across the spectrum from purely quantitative to purely qualitative data. Whilst not appropriate in all mixed methods research, this represents another way in which the researcher can potentially be creative in their approach to data collection.

In examining some of the research applications from various areas of research we wish to encourage the reader of this text to expand the traditional 'arsenal' of methods used in investigating health-related questions. The field of mixed methods research can innovatively combine a variety of data collection methods. The most common combination involves focus groups or interviews and quantitative surveys (for example, Chaboyer et al. 1998; Coyle and Williams 2000; Howarth and Kneafsey 2005) and individual interviews and (quasi-) experimental testing of interventions (Barlow et al. 2001). However, other innovative methods have been used with great promise, such as quantitative concept mapping, which involves both a qualitative and a quantitative element (Chun and Springer 2005). Some researchers have combined validated measures with in-depth interviews with success (Martin et al. 2003), while others used diaries and interviews (Ream et al. 2006). Others have applied a mixed methods approach to construct validation in cross-cultural research, in which findings from open responses in an ethnographic survey were used to validate the factorial structure of the quantitative portion of the survey (Hitchcock et al. 2005). This approach is useful in the development of quantitative data collection instruments that are culturally sensitive.

Interviews

Interviews are most commonly associated with qualitative research. However, they can be a useful tool in mixed methods research, either by providing qualitative data to be integrated with a quantitative dataset or by collecting mixed data. Whilst face-to-face interviews are perhaps the most common, other communications mediums such as telephones, email and Internet chat groups can be useful, particularly in geographically dispersed or isolated groups. Qualitative interviews can be an important addition to a survey or clinical trial in order to gain a deeper understanding or explanation of the quantitative findings (see Chapter 9). However, care must be taken to ensure that the interview data are collected for a specific purpose and appropriately integrated with the quantitative dataset rather than simply being a means to illustrate and add spice to the real results (Foss and Ellefsen 2002). As can be seen in the example of the study conducted by Jordan

Table 5.2 Data collection strategies (adapted from Johnson and Turner 2003; Halcomb and Davidson 2006).

	Pure qualitative	Mixed	Pure quantitative
Interviews/ focus groups	**Informal conversational interviews** Unstructured, exploratory, in-depth interviews, open-ended questions	**Interview guide approach** Topic areas pre-specified on an interview guide but the researcher may vary the wording or order of questions depending on the participant	**Standardised open-ended approach** Open-ended, pre-specified questions, neither the wording or order of questions is changed by the interviewer	**Scripted interviews** Fully structured interaction with identical questions for all participants, closed-ended questions
Questionnaires	**Open survey** All survey questions are exploratory, in-depth and open-ended	**Mixed survey** A combination of closed-ended and open-ended questions		**Structured survey** Highly structured survey form with all closed-ended questions
Tests	**Open instrument** All items require some degree of judgement by the rater. Definitions of these items are fairly broad	**Mixed instrument** A combination of items some of which require some judgement by the rater		**Structured instrument** Highly structured test with all closed-ended items. The definitions of the responses for each item are rigid
Observations	**Informal observations** Unstructured, exploratory, in-depth observations, open-ended questions	**Guided observation** Topic areas pre-specified on an observation guide but the researcher may vary the interaction in response to the participant	**Standardised observation** Pre-specified observation framework applied consistently by the observer	**Structured observation** Fully structured interaction with specific data collected using a pre-determined set of data items. All data items are defined prior to the observation
Secondary data	**Informal data collection** Unstructured, exploratory, in-depth observations of secondary sources. Open-ended questions may be used to direct data collection	**Guided data collection** Topic areas pre-specified on a data collection tool but the researcher may vary the data collected in response to the source data that emerges	**Standardised data collection** Pre-specified tool for data collection which is applied consistently by the data collector	**Structured data collection** Fully structured data collection with specific data collected using a pre-determined set of data items. All data items are clearly defined prior to commencing data collection

---

Box 5.1 Research in action

Jordan et al. (2006) interviewed 20 adults with long-term percutaneous endoscopic gastrostomies using both semi-structured and
structured approaches. Initially, qualitative data were collected
using a semi-structured interview process. Following this, quantitative data were collected via a symptom checklist adapted from
the gastro-intestinal quality of life instrument and an established
quality of life measure (Short Form 12). From analysis of the qualitative data it was evident that participants experienced a significant
'burden of treatment' related to their percutaneous endoscopic gastrostomies. However, it was only when the structured quantitative
data were examined that several important and treatable symptoms were revealed within the group. Identification of such
symptoms is vital for appropriate management strategies to be
implemented. Whilst the researchers identified some limitations in
the use of the Short Form 12 with this population group, the quantitative data that this and the symptom checklist provided were
invaluable in providing a comprehensive evaluation of the patients'
perspective of their percutaneous endoscopic gastrostomy.

---

et al. (2006), interviews can also be used to collect both qualitative and
quantitative data (see Box 5.1). Combining qualitative and quantitative
data collection has several advantages; in particular, both qualitative
and quantitative data will be available for the same participants,
missing quantitative data items will be minimised and data collection
can be achieved in a short timeframe. However, these advantages must
be balanced against the high participant burden created by the timeframe required to conduct such extensive data collection in a single
encounter.

Focus groups

Focus groups are an effective way of collecting qualitative data from a
group of persons who are familiar with the research problem. Focus
groups require a skilled group facilitator if they are to be successful
and it is better if the group is of a small to moderate size (Morgan 1998).
Focus groups can capture the particularities and breadth of opinions
about a topic. They also provide a context for observing social interaction and how opinions are arrived at. Focus groups can either generate
purely qualitative data regarding participants' opinions or experiences,
purely quantitative data such as priorities for action, or mixed data.
Table 5.3 provides some examples of how focus groups have been used
to date in mixed methods research.

Table 5.3 Use of focus groups in mixed methods research.

Reference	Design	Data collection	Findings
Davis and Miller (2006)	Concurrent triangulation	Focus groups Knowledge questionnaire	Focus group data revealed that few participants could accurately define glycaemic index or explain how it related to blood glucose levels. Questionnaire findings confirmed the focus group data regarding limited knowledge of the glycaemic index. During the focus groups participants identified methods of education that they would prefer. Such information provided direction in the subsequent development of education strategies
Stacey et al. (2005)	Sequential exploratory	Interviews with key informants Focus groups Simulated patient calls Survey	Stacey et al. (2005) sought to identify the barriers and facilitators influencing the provision of decision support by call centre nurses to callers facing values-sensitive health decisions at a Canadian province-wide health call centre. Key informant interviews, focus groups and simulated patient calls provided data to inform the development of the barriers assessment survey
Galantino et al. (2005)	Sequential explanatory	Randomised trial Focus groups Journals Non-participant observation	This randomised clinical trial investigated the effects of t'ai chi and aerobic exercise on functional outcomes and quality of life in patients with AIDS in two American outpatient infectious disease clinics. The primary quantitative outcomes included quality of life, functional measures, physical performance and psychological changes. To consider the patients' explanations for these measurements, qualitative data were collected from subjects' journals, focus groups and non-participant observation

Questionnaires

Survey administration represents a relatively cost-effective means of collecting data from a large sample in a short period of time (King et al. 2001; Fink 2003b). The perceived anonymity of respondents can be a significant advantage in terms of collecting information about participants' true feelings (Tashakkori and Teddlie 2003). Mixed methods designs can enhance the efficacy of survey research in two major ways. Firstly, various qualitative methods can inform development of the survey instrument (for example, Stacey et al. 2005). The use of closed-ended questions is an alluring strategy to simplify data analysis (Fink 2003a). Developing such questions from a preceding qualitative stage can increase the researchers' confidence that suitable options have been provided. Secondly, qualitative methods can be used to further explore either general or specific survey findings (for example, Halcomb 2005; Judd et al. 2006) (Box 5.2) or explain outlying or deviant cases (Barbour 1999).

Box 5.2 Research in action

Judd et al. (2006) examined the rate of mental health issues amongst farmers compared to non-farmer rural residents in an attempt to understand the increased risk of suicide amongst farmers. First they used self-report questionnaire data to compare rates of mental health problems (a common correlate of suicide) and a number of personality measures between farmers ($n = 371$) and non-farming rural residents ($n = 380$). Semi-structured interviews with farmers ($n = 32$) were then used to gain a richer understanding of how the contexts of farming and mental health interact.

Observation

Observation can also collect data across the continuum of qualitative–quantitative data. Observation using a highly structured checklist, for example, may be used for quantitative data collection. Whilst this type of observation may be conceptually appealing, care must be taken to establish inter-observer (rater) reliability if multiple observers are used to collect data. Observation seeking to collect qualitative data may be much less structured, with field notes taken by the researcher to record their observations and interviews with participants to explore observations (for example, Luck et al. 2008) (Box 5.3). While observation may be an effective method of data collection capturing events as they happen, observation can be time consuming and may require a researcher to spend long periods of time in the research setting collecting data.

Box 5.3 Research in action

In a doctoral project, Luck et al. (2008) used a variety of methods including structured and unstructured observation to explore the issue of violence in the emergency department. The observational tool which was developed specifically for the study was used to measure both structured observations and semi-structured contextual information. Other data collection methods included field notes and interviews with registered nurses. The meanings that nurses assigned to violent acts were found to influence their response to these acts of violence towards nurses by patients, and accompanying relatives or friends.

Practical issues in planning data collection

Balancing strengths and limitations

An important consideration in selecting data collection methods is the need to ensure that methods are combined in such a way that the limitations of one method are balanced by the strengths of another (Johnson and Onwuegbuzie 2004; Andrew and Halcomb 2006). For example, a major limitation of surveys is the lack of depth possible in closed-ended items. The addition of interviews with a subgroup of survey respondents can assist in enhancing the richness of data and explaining some of the survey findings (Box 5.4).

Timing of data collection

Several mixed methods designs call for a two-stage, sequential approach to data collection, whereby data collected during the first stage informs the subsequent data collection. We have observed that several of our research students have been impatient to move their projects along, without first fully analysing the data from the first stage and incorporating its findings into their subsequent plans for data collection. It is vital, when planning project timelines, that sufficient time and resources be given to this interim analysis to maximise the effectiveness of the design.

Box 5.4 Research in action

In the first phase of her doctoral project, Halcomb (2005) conducted a sequential exploratory study to examine the current role of the general practice nurse in Australia and their perceptions regarding the potential for role expansion related to chronic cardiovascular disease. Two hundred and eighty-four nurses responded to a national survey. Data from the survey provided demographic and employment characteristics and revealed some of the relationships between these characteristics and the practice nurses' role (Halcomb et al. 2008b). It became evident, however, that there was a mismatch between the number of participants who perceived that a particular task was appropriate and those who undertook the task in their practice. This mismatch was not completely explained by demographic or employment characteristics. Extrinsic factors such as legal and funding issues, lack of space and general practitioner attitudes were identified as barriers to role expansion. Although these barriers were identified, the researcher did not fully understand exactly how they impacted upon the nurse. Therefore, semi-structured interviews ($n = 10$) were conducted to clarify in detail how these barriers impacted upon the nurses' role in clinical practice (Halcomb et al. 2008a).

Plan for data analysis

Whilst data analysis is discussed in detail in Chapter 6, it is important that researchers consider how they will manage and analyse the various data that they are planning to collect. Consideration should also be given to the practicalities and potential value of integrating various datasets (Box 5.5). Attention to this during the planning phase is important to maximise the quality of the final data analysis and reporting.

Box 5.5 Point to ponder

Integrating qualitative and quantitative datasets during data analysis can, in many cases, provide a greater insight into the information that the data yields than would have been possible through analyses that only considered each dataset separately.

Sampling

Mixed methods research designs vary not only in terms of their purposes, the complexity of the design and phasing of the methods in the
research process, as has been discussed in Chapter 3, but also in the
sampling logic that they employ. Mixed methods research designs
often combine more than one sampling strategy.

Sampling is determined by theoretical and pragmatic considerations.
Researchers need to pay attention to resources that they have at their
disposal, which in turn are often determined by levels of funding. This
is not to say that research questions and designs need to be formulated
in order to meet budget and resource targets but there has to be a
balance between the feasibility and the necessity to conduct a study.
The objective has to be to obtain the best possible datasets, using the
most economical amount of resources. Table 5.4 provides sampling
criteria proposed by Curtis et al. (2000) which, although intended for
qualitative research, may be applied to any form of sampling.

This list of guidelines was expanded by Kemper et al. (2003) to
include the notion that 'the sampling plan should allow the research
team to transfer/generalize the conclusions of the study to other settings or populations' and 'the sampling scheme should be as efficient
as practical' (p. 276). Clearly, sampling has to be meaningful in that it
enables the researcher to answer a set of research questions within a
particular conceptual framework. The data that are collected need to
be of the best possible quality to allow for making credible inferences
and/or theoretical extrapolation. Unnecessary or extraneous data collection should be avoided since it places a burden on research participants and is probably violating privacy and data protection principles.
Also, the more data that are collected, the greater the analysis required.
This again may jeopardise the feasibility of the study. However, findings from one particular study are most useful if they have value
beyond the scope of the sample and particular study context, and if

Table 5.4 Sampling guidelines (Curtis et al. 2000: 1003).

The sampling strategy should stem logically from the conceptual framework as well as from the research questions being addressed by the study
The sample should be able to generate a thorough database on the type of phenomena under study
The sample should at least allow the possibility of drawing clear inferences from the data; the sample should allow for credible explanations
The sampling strategy must be ethical
The sampling plan should be feasible

results can be 'generalised' to a larger population or practice field. Finally, it is critical that researchers are judicious with the resources at their disposal. Research should not only be feasible and practical but its conduct needs to be efficient as well.

Currently, sampling strategies unique to mixed methods research do not exist. Sampling in mixed methods research usually relies on the combination of probability and non-probability sampling approaches that have traditionally been used in qualitative and quantitative research (Box 5.6).

Box 5.6 Point to ponder

Sampling is the term used to describe the process of selecting participants to 'represent' populations. Sampling strategies can be classified as either probability or non-probability. Probability sampling involves the random selection of participants from the population. Non-probability sampling (convenience, quota and purposive sampling) selects participants based on their characteristics.

Sampling in sequentially organised mixed methods studies frequently means that purposive samples are generated based on probability or another sampling component (QUAN–QUAL designs). For example, a survey has demonstrated that some individuals with particular coping strategies have better pain outcomes. The survey does not provide any information about how these coping strategies actually work, why they are chosen and how they have been acquired. Consequently, the researcher decides to examine the coping strategies of these particular individuals in greater detail and selects them purposively for qualitative in-depth interviews. In some cases, purposive samples that produce exploratory information provide researchers with a rationale for a stratified probability sampling approach (QUAL–QUAN designs). For example, the researcher may learn that age plays an important role in what format patients would like to receive medication information. Before starting the experimental component of the study, the researcher then decides to stratify the random sample by age groups.

Sample size considerations in mixed methods research are driven by the particular requirements for each study component. It is critical that quality standards (e.g. reliability, validity for quantitative methods, trustworthiness for qualitative methods) are not compromised due to the fact that the mixed methods study comprises of both qualitative and quantitative data collections.

The need for reflectivity in combining methods

As Hammersley (2005) identifies, the various rationales for conducting mixed methods research all make numerous assumptions. Thus just as seeking to corroborate data from different sources may not lead us down the path of validation, so too the complementarity rationale for mixing methods may not complete the picture either. There may be no meeting point between epistemological positions that underpin the use of different methods as in the use of data collected by researchers coming from different philosophical positions. However, as Hammersley (2005) suggests, there is a need for a dialogue between them. What is clear is that mixed methods research, if carried out in a technicist way, obviates the need for reflection about methods: 'these [different forms of triangulation] are investigative strategies that offer evidence to inform judgements, not techniques that provide guaranteed truth or completeness' (Hammersley 2005: 12).

Halfpenny (2005) cuts to the heart of some of the problems researchers seem to get into when they justify a combination of methods in terms of philosophical positions. He too challenges the assumption of a simple correspondence between philosophical position and research techniques. Rather there is a number of logics at play in formulating research questions, creating a research design, choosing methods and analysing data. These logics do not map on to one another neatly. Brannen stated in 1992 that data collected from different methods cannot simply be added together to produce a unitary or rounded reality or truth (Brannen 1992, Brannen 2005). For if we move away from assuming that we are trying to arrive at a single reality we need to understand how different accounts are arrived at and the purposes that these accounts serve (Hammersley 2005).

What needs to be kept in mind in combining methods is the relation between theory, methods and data. For example, a recent debate about apparently conflicting findings from two studies, one using qualitative and one quantitative methods, suggests that the issue is not only about methods (Anderson et al. 2005; Brannen and Nilsen 2007). The studies explored young people's ways of thinking about, and their plans for, the future. The theoretical propositions and conceptualisations that the researchers employed in these studies were very different and informed the kinds of questions they framed to young people and the research methods they chose. Not surprisingly they produced very different results (Anderson et al. 2005; Brannen and Nilsen 2007). These studies used different methods: one a large-scale quantitative survey and the other a cross-national qualitative study using focus groups and interviews. However, this is not to say that it might have been possible to formulate similar, though not exactly the same, questions to young people in both studies had the theoretical and conceptual formulations concerning the idea of 'planning' been similarly sensitive. In the qualitative study distinctions were made in such a way that plans were conceptualised as concrete and relating to the short term. By contrast hopes were less concrete and more aspirational, and related to the longer term. Dreams, on the other hand, were idealistic and belonged to a fantasy world. In the survey only one concept was used to cover all such possibilities. Yet both studies had set out to investigate variation in the ways in which young people thought about their futures and differences in meanings (Brannen and Nilsen 2007).

Conclusion

In this chapter we have provided many examples of mixed methods data collection to illustrate that there are many ways of achieving a mixing of methods. There is not a defined set of prescriptions for conducting mixed methods research. The researcher must clearly justify their use of particular methods for collecting data with reference to the research questions, theoretical frameworks and research designs of their studies.

The potential combinations of different methods of data collection within this genre of research is extensive. Methods of collecting data are often selected according the practicalities of what is feasible and possible to do given the resources available and the conditions for studying a particular phenomenon (Bryman 1984, Brannen 1992).

References

Anderson M., Bechhofer F., McCrone D., Jamieson L., Li Y. and Stewart R. (2005) Timespans and plans among young adults. *Sociology*, **39**, 139–155.

Andrew S. and Halcomb E.J. (2006) Mixed methods research is an effective method of enquiry for working with families and communities. *Contemporary Nurse*, **23**, 145–153.

Barbour R.S. (1999) The case for combining qualitative and quantitative approaches in health services research. *Journal of Health Services Research Policy*, **4**, 39–43.

Barlow J., Wright C. and Kroll T. (2001) Overcoming perceived barriers to employment among people with arthritis. *Journal of Health Psychology*, **6**, 205–216.

Brannen J. (1992) *Mixing Methods: Qualitative and Quantitative Research*. Aldershot: Avebury.

Brannen J. (2004) Working qualitatively and quantitatively in Seale C., Gobo G., Gubrium J.F. and Silvermon D. (eds.), *Qualitative Research Practice*, London: Sage.

Brannen J. (2005) Mixing methods: the entry of qualitative and quantitative approaches into the research process. *International Journal of Social Research Methodology*. Special Issue **8**(3), 173–185.

Brannen J. and Nilsen A. (2007) Young people, time horizons and planning: a response to Anderson et al. *Sociology*, **41**, 153–161.

Bryman A. (1984) The debate about quantitative and qualitative research: a question of method or epistemology. *British Journal of Sociology*, **35**, 76–92.

Chaboyer W., McMurray A. and Patterson E. (1998) Unlicensed assistive personnel in the critical care unit: What is their role? *International Journal of Nursing Practice*, **4**, 240–246.

Chun J. and Springer D.W. (2005) Stress and coping strategies in runaway youths: an application of concept mapping. *Brief Treatment and Crisis Intervention*, **5**, 57–74.

Constantino R., Crane P.A., Noll B.S., Doswell W.M. and Braxter B. (2007) Exploring the feasibility of email-mediated interaction in survivors of abuse. *Journal of Psychiatric and Mental Health Nursing*, **14**, 291–301.

Coyle J. and Williams B. (2000) An exploration of the epistemological intricacies of using qualitative data to develop a quantitative measure of user views of health care. *Journal of Advanced Nursing*, **31**, 1235–1243.

Curtis S., Gesler W., Smith G. and Washburn S. (2000) Approaches to sampling and case selection in qualitative research: examples in the geography of health. *Social Science and Medicine*, **50**, 1001–1014.

Davis M.S. and Miller C.K. (2006) Educational needs regarding the glycemic index in diabetes management. *Topics in Clinical Nutrition*, **21**, 17–25.

Drummond K., Pierce L.L., Steiner V. and Hicks B. (2007) Young females' perceived experience of caring for husbands with stroke. *Online Journal of Nursing Informatics*, **11**, www.eaa-knowledge.com/ojni/ni/11_2/drummond.htm.

Fink A. (2003a) *How to Ask Survey Questions*. Thousand Oaks, California: Sage Publications.

Fink A. (2003b) *The Survey Handbook*. Thousand Oaks, California: Sage Publications.

Foss C. and Ellefsen B. (2002) The value of combining qualitative and quantitative approaches in nursing research by means of method triangulation. *Journal of Advanced Nursing*, **40**, 242–248.

Galantino M.L., Shepard K., Krafft L., LaPerriere A., Ducette J., Sorbello A. et al. (2005) The effect of group aerobic exercise and T'ai chi on functional outcomes and quality of life for persons living with acquired immunodeficiency syndrome. *Journal of Alternative and Complementary Medicine*, **11**, 1085–1092.

Halcomb E.J. (2005) *Carving a Niche for Australian Practice Nurses in Chronic Heart Failure Management*. PhD thesis, School of Nursing, University of Western Sydney, Australia.

Halcomb E.J. and Davidson P.M. (2006) Is verbatim transcription of interview data always necessary? *Applied Nursing Research*, **19**, 38–42.

Halcomb E.J., Davidson P.M., Griffiths R. and Daly J. (2008a) Cardiovascular disease management: time to advance the practice nurse role? *Australian Health Review*, **32**, 44–55.

Halcomb E.J., Davidson P.M., Salamonson Y. and Ollerton R. (2008b) Nurses in Australian general practice: implications for chronic disease management. *Journal of Nursing and Healthcare of Chronic Illness*, in association with *Journal of Clinical Nursing*, **17**, 6–15.

Halfpenny P. (2005) *The Reflection between Quantitative and Qualitative Research*. Mixed Methods Workshop, ESRC, Research Methods Programme. Manchester, England.

Hammersley M. (2005) *Troubles with Triangulation*. Mixed Methods Workshop, ESRC, Research Methods Programme. Manchester, England.

Hitchcock J.H., Nastasi B.K., Dai D.Y., Newman J., Jayasena A., Bernstein-Moore R. et al. (2005) Illustrating a mixed-method approach for validating culturally specific constructs. *Journal of School Psychology*, **43**, 259–278.

Howarth M.L. and Kneafsey R. (2005) The impact of research governance in healthcare and higher education organizations. *Journal of Advanced Nursing*, **49**, 675–683.

Johnson B. and Turner L.A. (2003) Data collection strategies in mixed methods research. In Tashakkori A. and Teddlie C. (eds.) *Handbook of Mixed Methods in Social and Behavioral Research*, pp. 297–320. Thousand Oaks, California: Sage Publications.

Johnson B.R. and Onwuegbuzie A.J. (2004) Mixed methods research: a research paradigm whose time has come. *Educational Researcher*, **33**, 14–26.

Jordan S., Philpin S., Warring J., Cheung W.Y. and Williams J. (2006) Percutaneous endoscopic gastrostomies: the burden of treatment from a patient perspective. *Journal of Advanced Nursing*, **56**, 270–281.

Judd F., Jackson H., Fraser C., Murray G., Robins G. and Komiti A. (2006) Understanding suicide in Australian farmers. *Social Psychiatry and Psychiatric Epidemiology*, **41**, 1–10.

Kemper E., Stringfield S. and Teddlie C. (2003) Mixed methods sampling strategies in social science research. In Tashakkori A. and Teddlie C. (eds.) *Handbook of Mixed Methods in Social and Behavioral Research*, pp. 273–296. Thousand Oaks, California: Sage Publications.

King K.A., Pealer L.N. and Bernard A.L. (2001) Increasing response rates to mail questionnaires: a review of inducement strategies. *American Journal of Health Education*, **32**, 4–15.

Luck L., Jackson D. and Usher K. (2008) Innocent or culpable? Meanings that emergency department nurses ascribe to individual acts of violence. *Journal of Clinical Nursing*, **17**, 1071–1078.

Martin L., Farrell M., Lambrenos K. and Nayagam D. (2003) Living with the Ilizarov frame: adolescent perceptions. *Journal of Advanced Nursing*, **43**, 478–487.

McEvoy P. and Richards D. (2006) A critical realist rationale for using a combination of quantitative and qualitative methods. *Journal of Research in Nursing*, **11**, 66–78.

Morgan D.L. (1998) *The Focus Group Guidebook*. Thousand Oaks, California: Sage Publications.

Ream E., Gibson F., Edwards J., Seption B., Mulhall A. and Richardson A. (2006) Experience of fatigue in adolescents living with cancer. *Cancer Nursing*, **29**, 317–326.

Stacey D., Graham I.D., O'Connor A.M. and Pomey M.-P. (2005) Barriers and facilitators influencing call centre nurses' decision support for callers facing values-sensitive decisions: a mixed methods study. *Worldviews on Evidence-Based Nursing*, **2**, 184–195.

Tashakkori A. and Teddlie C. (eds.) (2003) *Handbook of Mixed Methods in Social and Behavioral Research*. Thousand Oaks, California: Sage Publications.

Analysing Mixed Methods Data

Patricia Bazeley

Learning objectives

After reading this chapter, you will have the knowledge to:

a) Identify and evaluate strategies used for combining data from multiple sources in published literature.
b) Explore possibilities in mixed methods data analysis beyond separate reporting of statistical outcomes and 'emergent themes'.
c) Design strategies to enrich data analyses in your own research.

Introduction

My contextual starting point for this chapter is the need to move beyond current practice, but the primary focus of the chapter is on strategies for analysis in mixed methods research. In reviewing these, I move from strategies which involve working separately with different forms of data for corroboration, development or expansion to those in which qualitative and quantitative data are synthesised or combined for analysis. I then review those strategies which involve conversion of data from one form to another, and application of multiple forms of analysis to the same dataset. Illustrative examples from the published literature are provided for each strategy. Where relevant, I explain the potential contribution of computer software in facilitating analysis. Because analysing data occurs in a context of project philosophy and design, I also review key issues of epistemology and integration as they apply to data analysis when mixing methods.

Analysing mixed methods data generally assumes competence in analysing, separately, both quantitative (statistical) and qualitative (textual) data. No attempt is made, in this chapter, to develop these specific competencies. Rather, the objective is to stimulate thinking about more effective ways to apply these skills in making use of the multiple data sources you may have gathered, to genuinely integrate the findings of these, and to provide some practical guidance on how this might be done so that you can enrich the analyses you undertake.

The context – current practice

Employment of mixed methods has become fashionable in health services and nursing research. There is now an extensive range of literature in which health researchers report using multiple data sources with the expressed purpose of seeking convergence in results from different sources for validation, or to provide complementary data in order to enrich their conclusions. The majority, however, are treating these differently shaped data as entirely separate components of their study, with some going so far as to publish them in separate articles (O'Cathain et al. 2007). Others focus more on the theoretical benefits of mixing than on their practice of it (Kinn and Curzio 2005). Bryman (2007) noted that many mixed methods researchers experienced difficulty in 'bringing together the analysis and interpretation of the quantitative and the qualitative data and writing a narrative that linked the analyses and interpretations' (p. 10). While these strategies for handling mixed data may sometimes be appropriate to the purpose of the study and publication restrictions can encourage separate reporting of different components, often the lack of integration represents significant lost opportunities for a far richer, deeper analysis of the available data.

Integration and analysis purposes

Many researchers believe that it is necessary to first derive results from separate qualitative and quantitative component studies before those results can be drawn together and interpreted as mixed methods data (Sale et al. 2002; Morse 2003). Moran-Ellis et al. (2006) referred to this approach as theoretical integration, preferring to reserve the term 'integration' for mixed methods studies where combination occurs from the point of conceptualisation through all phases of the research.

For others, integration of qualitative and quantitative approaches might occur at any stage throughout a mixed methods study (Creswell 2003; Maxwell and Loomis 2003; Yin 2006). Moran-Ellis et al. (2006) argued that integration requires equal weight be given to each approach and that the approaches used are interdependent in building a coherent whole in the service of a particular research purpose. The use of a combination of approaches at every stage of a study should be a matter of general principle, in Yin's (2006) view. He argued, for example, for the use of both qualitative and quantitative data and analysis methods in addressing aspects of both process and outcome in an evaluation study rather than the more usual practice of using quantitative measures of outcome and qualitative approaches to assess process. At the very least, mixed methods research should be analysed, interpreted and reported 'in such a way that the quantitative and qualitative components are mutually illuminating' (Bryman 2007: 8).

In their early review of 57 mixed methods evaluation articles, Greene et al. (1989) found only five studies in which analyses were integrated prior to final interpretation and conclusions. Strategies for integration identified in those five studies served a primary purpose of initiation, that is, to gain 'fresh insights and new perspectives that enhance conceptual understanding' (Caracelli and Greene 1993: 203). Similarly, in his review of 232 mixed methods projects across a range of disciplines, Bryman (2006) identified relatively few studies which demonstrated integration of different data forms or analytical procedures in the analysis phase.

Dichotomising approaches to research 'masks the reality that there can be many different "mixes" or combinations of methods' including, for example, the combination of experiment and survey, survey and case study (Yin 2006: 41). Not only is it impossible to entirely distinguish qualitative and quantitative approaches, but such a distinction is less than useful when approaching analysis (Coxon 2005). 'Qualitative' and 'quantitative' have been compared on at least 30 different dimensions, so that they are best viewed as the ends of a multidimensional continuum, with any one study potentially being located at different points across that continuum for each dimension (Bazeley 2004). 'Ultimately all methods of data collection are analysed "qualitatively", in so far as the act of analysis is an interpretation, and therefore of necessity a selective rendering, of the "sense" of the available data'

(Fielding and Fielding 1986: 12). Integration of data and/or approaches to analysis is a logical consequence of such a view.

Critically, analytical strategies, particularly decisions about the level of integration in mixed methods studies and the point at which it might occur, are very much related to issues of research design and purpose. Bryman (2006) noted a weak link generally between purpose and methods in mixed methods studies. Greene et al. (1989) observed muddled use of terms (particularly triangulation) and noted a need to think through carefully planned and defensible rationales for mixed methods studies (see also Chapter 4). Congruence between purpose and analysis is a critical feature in Maxwell and Loomis' (2003) interactive model of mixed methods design. Maxwell and Loomis (2003) observed that difficulty in identifying the extent of and approach to integration of qualitative and quantitative components in a study is often compounded by discrepancies between the asserted purposes and design of the study and the actual conduct of the study. They see the purpose and questions for the study as the primary driver for methods choices, including analysis strategies and approach to integration.

Philosophical assumptions and approaches to analysis

Three alternative strategies are presented to the mixed methods data analyst with regard to resolving issues raised by the possibility that the different approaches they are taking may be based on conflicting paradigmatic (ontological and epistemological) positions:

- Where the different components of a mixed methods study are seen as having different philosophical bases, keep the data gathering and analyses for each component separate until final integration of the separately developed results. This argument is epistemologically flawed, however, because if different methods are used then logically you can't combine information based on incompatible assumptions any more than you can combine the methods.
- Conduct the different components (data, analyses) from within a common philosophical basis, so that integration can occur at any stage. Most often, the philosophical bases chosen under these circumstances will be pragmatism or critical realism.
- Deliberately employ a dialectical combination of paradigms as a way to initiate fresh ideas and knowledge.

The belief that there is an essential link between a particular method-ological approach, or use of a particular type of data, and a particular paradigmatic viewpoint remains implicit in many mixed methods studies in nursing and the health sciences despite being broadly dis-missed in the literature. This belief was challenged by Morgan (2007) as being unsustainable as it is tied to a metaphysical view of what constitutes a research paradigm. In accepting Kuhn's preferred view of paradigms as currently accepted practices within a particular com-munity of scholars, Morgan (2007) argued for the appropriateness, for the community of mixed methods researchers, of a pragmatic view of methodology and methods in which a selected methodology (condi-tioned by the research question) is the primary determinant of both epistemology and methods.

In so far as quantitative and qualitative approaches are 'inextric-ably intertwined' at all levels of design, data collection and analysis, the real issue is more to do with whether the researcher is taking an analytical (controlled) or a systemic (complexity) approach. 'The ques-tion, then, is not whether the two sorts of data and associated methods can be linked during study design, but whether it should be done, how it will be done, and for what purposes' (Miles and Huberman 1994: 41).

Strategies for analysis

In reviewing particular strategies for analysis of mixed methods data, I move from those strategies in which the data and the analyses are kept *separate* until the point of conclusion and discussion, through *combining data types* for synthesis or comparison, to strategies which involve *mixing approaches to analysis* of data, typically involving conver-sion from one form to another. Finally I review some strategies that don't fit neatly into any of those boxes!

Separate data and analyses

The most common purposes for which separate substudies are designed are triangulation, complementarity/expansion, or development. When separate collection and analyses of quantitative and qualitative data occur before the two datasets are drawn together for discussion, there would appear to be no special mixed methods analysis strategies required. There are, nevertheless, at least three analysis issues to consider:

- The (relative) quality of each of the separate analyses.
- How the results of the separate analyses are to be synthesised in order to draw conclusions that incorporate both sets of data.
- Strategies to manage findings that are contradictory rather than complementary.

Triangulation

Triangulation is a much used and abused term (Barbour 1998; Andrew and Halcomb 2006). Although originally employed in the context of validating conclusions through seeking confirmatory evidence from at least two sources (Greene et al. 1989), it is now also widely used to include the practice of seeking data from at least two sources with complementary strengths and non-overlapping weaknesses, such that data from one source complements or extends the other (Sandelowski 1995; Erzberger and Kelle 2003; Moran-Ellis et al. 2006). Given triangulation for completeness involves a more integrative approach to drawing conclusions from data, and therefore has more in common with complementarity, my preference is to reserve the term triangulation for confirmatory studies.

Whenever the purpose of the researcher in using more than one method is for corroboration or convergence of results, then both data gathering and analysis for each method is necessarily conducted separately, although usually concurrently. Pertinent results are identified within each method, confidence established in those, and then criteria (informed by existing knowledge, the purpose of the study and a desire to avoid weaknesses) for including those results in an integrated model are developed (Foster 1997). Thus it is only after the analyses have been completed that an assessment is made regarding the level of convergence in the results, with conclusions drawn based on all sets of data.

In their research on symptom experience associated with the development of acute rejection after lung transplantation, DeVito Dabbs et al. (2004) considered both physiological and interpretive responses so as to better identify points for preventive intervention. Patient reporting of symptoms via questionnaire was compared with results of clinical assessment of pulmonary infection and acute rejection through, for example, shortness of breath, cough and biopsy evidence. Additionally, interviews, phone calls, clinical records, field notes and memos were used in a grounded theory approach with a smaller, purposively selected sample to build a model ('striving for normalcy') which identified stages related to progressive sophistication in symptom response. Findings from both approaches were assembled to generate final conclusions. While DeVito Dabbs et al. (2004) saw the physiological and reporting components as being quantitative, and the interpretive responses as a qualitative component (appearing somewhat as an 'add on' to the main study), one might also read a patient's reporting of their symptoms as *their interpretation* of the physiological symptoms. With that perspective, mixed methods triangulation as confirmation can be seen to be occurring within that 'quantitative' component of the study.

McKeon et al. (2006) used survey data to build a path model showing how organisational variables contribute to potentially unsafe medication administration. Qualitative comments sought in the questionnaire supported conclusions drawn from the quantitatively derived model, and additionally pointed to why providing information is not effective in changing practice – with neither time nor readily available computers, information will not be accessed. Similarly, Flensner and Lindencrona (2002), in a quasi-experimental design, found that interview data supported scaled and diary data indicating that cooling suits bring multifaceted benefits for reducing fatigue in patients with multiple sclerosis. The diaries and interviews, additionally, provided information on the specifics of how the suits worked to reduce fatigue.

These latter studies illustrate how confirmation and completeness, as goals of triangulation, may become conflated so that a particular study ends up incorporating both (Coyle and Williams 2000). It behoves the researcher to make clear which of these purposes is intended, although, as noted by Maxwell and Loomis (2003), methods tend not to remain as separate in practice as design theory would suggest.

Expansion or complementarity

Expansion or complementary designs employ one method to explain, extend or compensate for the other. In these most common of mixed methods designs (Bryman 2006), data might be gathered either concurrently or sequentially. Again, the analyses are usually undertaken separately with integration occurring at the point at which results are being discussed and conclusions drawn.

Complementary approaches are typically employed in evaluation studies where the focus tends to be on using quantitative data to measure outcomes and qualitative methods to understand the processes by which the outcomes are achieved. For example, interview data provided Schrijnemaekers et al. (2002) with an explanation as to why an attempt to strengthen emotion-orientated care in psychogeriatric facilities had produced no measurable change. The interviews with staff complemented post-intervention observations of their interactions with patients and analysis of case notes, each of which had indicated no comparative pattern of difference between intervention and control sites in patterns of care.

Gathering both quantitative and qualitative data is of benefit, also, in experimental research, to understand complex interventions (Polit and Hungler 1991). Simons (2007) conducted case studies of community mental health nurses' experience of involvement in a randomised controlled trial of different models of intervention with patients. Again, she was able to point out the difficulties experienced by those who have to implement procedures for a strictly controlled trial. Although this data complemented and helped to explain trial outcomes, Simons (2007) noted that she felt constrained to bracket her earlier experience of overseeing implementation of the trial when thinking about and analysing the interviews with the trial nurses.

In both the evaluation and experimental trial studies, then, analysis of complementary interview data helped to identify not just why an intervention was effective or not, but also the ways in which the conduct of the intervention itself may have been less 'pure' than was intended.

Expansionary designs do not always involve such distinct separation of data. In a study of patient participation in health care interviews described by Jones and Bugge (2006), interviews with clinicians were combined with conversation analysis (CA) of videotaped observations and follow-up think-aloud protocols with patients to provide a more complete picture of difficulties in participation. Each instance of difficulty in participation became the 'case' for additional analysis. In the case analysis, clinician and patient interviews extended the information gained through CA of particular events, but also CA provided necessary focus for the follow-up interviews. Thus, for example:

> . . . in this case the patient disregarded an opportunity to participate in the consultation (made apparent through CA and the addition of an 'external analyst') by withholding her views about the effectiveness of rods as a method of contraception. She did not want to disclose information that related to her friend (made apparent through think aloud), a situation (withholding information) which the nurse previously acknowledged (in interviews) as sometimes occurring at the professional's behest, not the patient's, in certain contexts during family planning consultations (Jones and Bugge 2006: 615).

Development

When one method is used as a tool in the development of the other, analysis of data gathered using different methods will be sequential, but there is a level of integration 'on the way' as the results of the first method will inform the design and analysis of the second (Caracelli and Greene 1993). Most often this strategy is employed in designing a quantitative instrument based on analysis of qualitative interview or focus group data, but it may also be used, for example, to identify a sample (or issues) for further investigation following a quantitative study.

Preliminary focus groups and then a nominal group technique were used by Ginsburg et al. (2005) to assist their design of a quantitative survey about things that influence parental control of type 1 diabetes in their children. From these they generated 30 items that reflected parents' priorities, expressed in their own language, rather than the views and language of the clinicians. Statistical results of the survey were presented with comparative analyses for different demographic and disease groups for each of the 30 questions. These results were then integrated with insights from the preliminary group meetings and from follow-up interviews conducted with 67 of the 799 parents who had responded to the survey in a discussion based around six key themes.

In their study of at-risk sexual behaviour and AIDS, Nickel et al. (1995), used cluster analysis with the results of a brief quantitative survey to generate eight clusters of sexually active 14–24-year-old youths. A sample for detailed interviews was drawn from two low-risk and three high-risk clusters of the sexually active youths. They first chose those who were most typical of their cluster, and then randomly selected from those who remained after 'not really fitting' cases were eliminated. The preliminary survey was necessary to identify an appropriate population of youths from which to draw for the primary qualitative component of the study.

Analysis of contradictory or discrepant results

When separate analyses give rise to contradictory or discrepant results, the researcher will usually attempt to propose an explanation to reconcile the discrepancy. Resolving the puzzle may result in a methodological explanation, or alternatively in fresh insights relating to the substantive issues (Mathison 1988). The researcher searches for a logical pattern, rather like piecing together a puzzle in a manner which is more like an overall qualitative approach (Jick 1979). While Jick (1979) considers that 'qualitative data and analysis function as the glue that cements the interpretation of multimethod results' (p. 609), others are more inclined to dismiss conflicting qualitative results (Patton 1988).

Meetoo and Temple (2003) used interviews and diary records to assess diabetics' adherence to diet. The interviews allowed them to classify the participants as being strict, moderately or very flexible with respect to controlling their diet. While there were many points of overlap between the interview and diary data, there were some for whom the data differed, for example where they indicated a strict attitude to diet, but had multiple diary examples of non-adherence. From this they generated a discussion about how the way in which people view and report self-care is related to context: in their study, for some the interview was confrontational and so they said the right thing, while for others, the diary was a permanent record, and so they wrote the right thing.

Resolving conflicting evidence between the two datasets often leads the researcher to construct new hypotheses. Although Erzberger and Kelle (2003) argue that these new explanations should be tested in a new study with new data, this is rarely reported in the literature.

Combining data types for synthesis

In keeping qualitative and quantitative data and analyses separate, particularly in complementary and expansion designs where there is no absolute need for separation, significant opportunities for enriching the analysis through earlier integration of the data are lost. Rather, Brewer and Hunter (2006) recommend 'a creative and at times even playful meshing of data-collecting methods to encourage serendipity and openness to new ideas' (p. 69).

Applying a common conceptual framework to varied data sources is an important first element in synthesising data at a group level. A combination of concurrent responses to the General Well Being scale and interview data was used by Hildebrandt and Kelber (2005) to evaluate the positive and negative impacts of work-based programmes for women on welfare. They coded the interview data using the same six constructs as are present in the General Well Being scale and also categorised the direction of change evident in the interviews for each construct as positive or negative, so that they could directly compare the scaled scores with the direction of the text responses in reviewing their results. In reporting their results they brought information together from both sources, including numerical data and illustrative text examples, relating to each construct. Beringer et al. (2006), similarly, used three concepts from Giddens' structuration theory (allocative resources, authoritative resources, rules) to guide coding and reporting of data from questionnaires, interviews, observations and documents on the issue of coordination of children's inpatient health care. From this, they arrived at the conclusion that care was diverse and inconsistent and was governed by tacit and informal rules.

Data are often gathered and recorded only on a group basis, yet where there is the possibility of finer-level matching of data, there exists opportunity for a fine-tuned synthesis or comparison, or even blending of different forms of data. The use of a tabular layout, referred to variously as a matrix or metamatrix (Miles and Huberman 1994; Happ et al. 2006), is a way to bring together varied data sources for particular cases or groups of cases. Table 6.1 provides an example where family case data about childhood immunisation, gathered through an interview and/or a questionnaire with the mother, have been tabulated using Excel and then sorted so that patterns for sub-groups might be more easily observed.

In her work on the effectiveness of therapeutic touch in controlling anxiety and pain in people requiring venipuncture, Wendler (2001) used a metamatrix to synthesise data following initial separate ana-lyses. This provided her with 'a secondary opportunity to determine if patterning exists that was not captured through compartmentalization into the quantitative or qualitative data analyses. Further, by using the meta-matrix, spontaneous comments and naturalistic events may be captured and considered within the context of the case' (Wendler 2001: 523). This led to the discovery of several unexpected relationships, including the discovery that participants and therapists reflected each others' language, often using identical words, and in so doing provided evidence of communication.

Meta-analysis and systematic review of mixed studies

Strategies for data synthesis can be applied not only to multiple sources of data within a study, but also to results and conclusions drawn from multiple studies. Such studies may be called for in the context of evidence-based practice or in expectation of a systematic review of previous research by funding bodies (Harden and Thomas 2005). The synthesis of results from differently conducted studies is achieved in ways reflective of the processes used in synthesising different forms of data, that is, using separate, sequential or integrated analyses (Sandelowski et al. 2006). Integration avoids the issue of classifying studies as qualitative or quantitative in the first place, but it often requires transformation of data in some form, in order to 'marry' diverse sources. Sandelowski et al. (2006) provide examples of quanti-fying qualitative results in order to be able to combine them with quantitative data and calculate effect sizes. In contrast, Harden and

Table 6.1 Partial matrix providing case comparison on experience of and attitudes to immunisation (Bazeley, unpublished data).

Case	Education	Age at last immunisation (mths)	Mention of needles, pain	Main thoughts re immunisation	Trusting	Questioning
Wendy	sc	12	Child cried	It will hurt and she'll cry	1	0
Felicity	sc	12	Fear of pain	Important, but fear of pain	1	0
Vivien	sc	18	Mother hates needles	Needles, but has to be done	1	1
Helen	sc	18	Tense, fear of pain	Fear of pain	1	0
Margie	sc	50+	Screams and kicking	Upset children, fear of needles	0	1
Kirstie	sc	50+	Child getting upset	Child getting upset	2	1
Susan	sc	50+	Fear of needle, upset	Child getting upset	1	0
Janice	hsc	Not immunised	No mention	Risk of reactions higher than risk of diseases	0	2
Sandra	hsc	1	No mention	Prevention of disease	1	1
Sue	hsc	18	No mention	Possible reaction	1	1
Angela	uni	1	Fearful beforehand	Protection from disease	1	2
Barbara	uni	6	No mention	Keep child healthy	2	0
Peta	uni	6	No mention	Possible side effects	3	1

sc: school certificate   hsc: higher school certificate   uni: university degree

Thomas (2005) recommend and provide an example of using the analytical themes they derived from qualitative 'views' data as a basis for organising categorised (i.e. qualitised) information extracted from quantitative 'trials' sources.

As is the case for synthesis of different data sources, if integration of the results and conclusions from differently conducted studies is to be achieved, a common conceptual framework is needed, and the use of a metamatrix tool, with or without transformation of particular components of data, would seem to be a most viable strategy for achieving the goal.

Combining data for comparative and pattern analysis

Placement of data into a common matrix or database allows for more than synthesis. Making comparisons is a basic strategy for analysis in almost any method. Comparisons facilitate a variety of outcomes, including: identification of subgroup characteristics; showing the behavioural or ideational correlates of scaled scores; showing the pattern of relationships between different constructs or variables; discernment of new dimensions within or related to a concept; validation of scale scores; and identification of outlier or deviant cases for further analysis (Bazeley 2006, 2007).

The most straightforward form of comparative or pattern analysis is when some aspect of the qualitative data is compared for demographic or other categorically or numerically defined subgroups of the sample. Although this can be done simply on a group average basis, ideally the analysis is based on data that were entered and therefore linked for individual cases, with the cases then sorted to reveal any patterns and discrepancies in the associated data. Even with a small sample, use of demographic or standardised scaled information can help to place in context what is said by a participant (Sandelowski 2000).

Benefits for understanding health care issues derived from combining scaled measures with narrative data on an individual respondent basis were reported by Kanzaki et al. (2004). Working with 12 female rheumatoid arthritis patients, Kanzaki et al. (2004) found that by 'combining a graphic representation of pain, mood and activity scores with patient narratives', they 'could identify the changes in coping and coping strategies in conjunction with changes in symptoms' (p. 233). Some of the women reported coexisting positive and negative coping, a finding which would not have been apparent through the use of standard coping scales alone.

The frustration of lost potential

In so many studies the researchers have multiple sources of data available for each participant, but they do not integrate these to compare responses and so leave many questions unanswered and possibilities for deeper insights unexplored. Indeed, within the nursing and health sciences literature, it was difficult to find clear examples where such integration, even just for comparative purposes, had been undertaken. For example, in a study of maternal vigilance by Carey et al. (2002), combination of scale with text data on an individual basis may have illuminated why there were some discrepancies between different sources of data and perhaps even why there were no real differences found in levels of vigilance between mothers of normal children and those whose child had a heart defect.

Martin et al. (2003) similarly had a rich array of physiological and scaled data for each participant in their study of adolescents living with an Ilizarov frame for skeletal adjustment. Again, the researchers did not connect these with their thematic analyses of interview data on an individual basis, and so they lost much of the potential benefit of the data they had available. A more integrative comparative analysis may also have helped them better explain why both resignation and social support were more evident in qualitative than quantitative responses.

Long-term survivors of lung cancer who scored lower in terms of distressed mood spoke more positively as a group about five central themes of existential issues, health and self-care, physical ability, adjustment and support (each described in detail) than did those who scored higher on distress (Maliski et al. 2003). While this information may be useful, the authors matched on a group basis only, ignored physiological measures such as spirometry results, even though these were described in detail in the method, and ignored a clear association of depression scores with racial and educational differences. A comparison of their five central themes based on these variables may have led them to entirely different conclusions.

Strategies and tools for comparison

Strategies for comparative analysis, beyond intuitively assessing separated piles of verbatim quotes, range from using hand-drawn matrices with summary data, through use of spreadsheets and databases, to the use of specialised quantitative or qualitative data analysis software. For strategies and tools relying on data being recorded in table-based format, it is usually necessary to work with summary (reduced) data, while comparison based on full text is more usual when qualitative analysis software is used. Software for analysis of qualitative data has replaced the need to create piles of cut-up documents on the lounge room floor, and offers significantly more flexibility in working with data than manual methods, including the capacity to ask many more, and more complex, questions of the data.

For a matrix, database or spreadsheet to be effective, data for each row must represent a case, with all the information (whether numbers, categories or text summaries or samples) for that case entered in that row (Table 6.1). A case might be an individual, but could also be a group, an event, a site, an article or document. Whatever it is, the case acts as the unit of analysis and provides the essential link between the different elements of data that have been gathered in relation to that case. Columns in the matrix are used to identify the different elements of data gathered, with their content determined by a combination of data type and conceptual framework. On occasions, the same information might be entered in two forms, being categorised in one column, and with summary or illustrative text samples in another. Typically some prior analysis of the qualitative data will have occurred in order to generate the particular elements to be considered, and to create the summary information for each case.

The simple (hand-drawn) matrix

In the hand-filled matrix, such as those popularised by Miles and Huberman (1994), it is necessary to sort the data before it is entered, in order to facilitate the detection of patterns. Thus, for example, to look at the impact of years of experience on the quality of care offered, columns would be created for recording information about each criterion for judging quality of care, and the data in the rows would be ordered by years of experience. The latter might initially be entered on a case-by-case basis, but depending on the number of cases, would then probably need to be grouped in order to interpret any patterns. As all other data would be ignored for this matrix, a fresh one would need to be created to consider, say, the role of hours of work in relation to quality of care.

When older people with dementia are admitted to acute nursing wards, it is important for nurses to be aware of their dementia and to take account of it in their care. Tolson et al. (1999) interviewed older patients with dementia and their main visitors using a critical incident technique, seeking positive aspects of care. 'Simple data matrices' were used to integrate the data from interviews with data from an audit of nursing records, from which they found that positive experiences of care were associated with documented care which addressed both the acute problem and the dementia.

Databases and spreadsheets

Databases and spreadsheets not only allow for the entry of numerical, categorical and text data within the same database, but they also provide tools for comparison and thus the examination of trends or discernment of patterns through their capacity to sort and re-sort data (Bazeley 2006, Niglas 2007). In that sense, then, they can be more efficient and effective than hand-drawn matrices. To start with, all the data for each case can be entered in a single matrix, with the cases entered in any order. Sort the data one way, learn what you can from that, then sort another way, or with a secondary variable. Examine the emerging patterns, and record what you have learned. Then, if you decide as part of the analysis you want to categorise the entries in a text column so that they too can be used as a basis for sorting against another column, it is a simple matter to add an additional column 'on the fly' to record those. Autofiltering options, split screens and pivot tables (cross-tabulations of categorical or scaled variables) may provide additional analytical assistance (Niglas 2007), while graphs generated from the data provide a visual display for analysis or presentation (Happ et al. 2006).

In a study of family coping with a child's chronic illness, Knafl and Ayres (1996) used a database to bring together summary data from interviews for different family members. Initial exploratory coding of a large volume of text data generated conceptual categories. Case summaries were prepared from each interview and coding from these was entered in the database in such a way that the focus on the family unit could be preserved while combining data from several sources. As they sorted data on family management style, for example, they were able to see patterns and check inconsistencies. Thus, they found a relationship between family management style and the constellation of family members' views of the child's illness. Because this technique is reductionist, they recommended its use at the end of an analysis, suggesting that 'early reliance on matrices over raw data or case summaries risks premature closure of the analysis and the development of overly simplistic descriptions and conceptualisations' (Knafl and Ayres 1996: 363).

Qualitative software

Qualitative data analysis software, such as NVivo, MaxQDA or Atlas.ti, allows the researcher to work with full text or summary notes (or other types of sources), using a priori or emergent categories to index (code) the content of the texts. Matching demographic, categorical or scaled data can be linked to the texts either on a case basis (NVivo) or a document basis (MaxQDA, Atlas.ti). This allows for rapid sorting of the coded text (for example, for a single concept or category, or for a number of related concepts) by the values of a variable. The resulting matrix can reveal if there are broad patterns of association between those values and presence of particular concepts in the textual data, and also if there are more subtle differences in forms of expression of a category across subgroups (Bazeley 2006, 2007). Each alternative component of the information provided (numbers, text) adds to the analytical picture: how many report and how they report might each be conditioned by (or associated with) the subgroup to which each case (or source) belongs. For example, mothers with incomplete high school education make reference to needles and crying when outlining their main thoughts about immunisation whereas those with more education typically refer to medical issues (Bazeley, unpublished data).

Ong et al. (2006) used NVivo to sort coded text from free responses about how life has been over the last 12 months at the end of a questionnaire about lower back pain (the final one in a 12-month series) and to compare coded responses to answers to comparable fixed response questions. Their use of odds ratios to compare responses to the two types of questions was unusual, but effective. They were able to determine through this procedure, for example, that when people talked freely about pain in various parts of their bodies, they did not, however, attribute pain in places other than the legs (for example, upper back, extremities) to their lower back problems.

In her doctoral study of nurses' care of patients who use illicit drugs, Ford (2006) used a combination of Stata and NVivo to analyse closed- and open-ended responses to a survey instrument. She found that the 311 of the 1605 respondents who wrote in free text responses about the interpersonal constraints these patients imposed on their therapeutic nursing role were more likely than others to be in high contact (i.e. clinical) areas of practice and reported more episodes of extended care for patients who were illicit drug users. They were also younger and less experienced than the remainder of the study sample, and while they reported higher levels of role adequacy, they also reported lower motivation and satisfaction. The specific therapeutic concerns they expressed were about patient aggressiveness, manipulation and irresponsibility, and they reported frustration with the patient, fear in their role and pessimism about the usefulness of therapeutic interventions. Within each of these more general categories, those from different practice groups expressed unique challenges which required different nursing care and which engendered different attitudes. Midwives dealt with manipulative patients and aggressive partners, but were particularly concerned about and frustrated with mothers' irresponsibility in the context of 'putting a baby in the mix';

for those working in emergency, attitudes to those seeking care were impacted by the short-term nature of a relationship in which they frequently experienced aggression and manipulation, were angered by irresponsibility toward others harmed by the drug users' actions, and where they did not see any long-term outcomes for the patient from the experience or their care; while for those in a medical/surgical practice setting, patients' aggressive and manipulative behaviour over an extended period of time-intensive contact created specific staffing and care issues.

Transforming data during analysis

Moving beyond combination of mixed data types to mixing approaches during data analysis typically involves conversion of data from one form to another. This might involve manipulation of a single set of data, or alternatively it occurs to facilitate the combination of qualitative and quantitative data from different sources.

Qualitising numerical data

At its simplest level, qualitising data might comprise nothing more than using scores to provide a descriptive classification of a sample. Going further, Tashakkori and Teddlie (1998: 130–133) described five kinds of narrative or qualitative profiling: modal, average, comparative, normative and holistic. While modal and average are descriptive, comparative and normative profiling are likely to be based on cluster or factor analyses. They illustrate with an example drawn from a study in which couples seeking marital therapy were grouped into five types based on clustering of responses to a personality inventory, and then verbally profiled in the context of marital therapy. Nickel et al. (1995) described different groups of sexually active youth in narrative terms on the basis of clusters of quantitative data, before sampling some of these groups for more 'in-depth' qualitative data.

Happ et al. (2006) provided an example where they qualitised scaled data in order to combine it in a matrix with other qualitative information on key dimensions derived from interviews and observations, in a study of medication taking among community-dwelling patients with dementia and their caregivers. The scaled data, such as from the mini-mental status examination, was reduced to categories (high, medium, low) and the qualitative comments or observations were entered as summary text along with a rating (for example, data for cooperation for one patient was entered as directable, doesn't resist, requires repeat cues and was classified as moderate; another was entered as reminds caregiver to refill and was classified as high). Sorting of the dataset is then possible based on any categorised concept or variable.

In her book on narrative analysis, Elliott (2005) devoted two chapters to the possibility of developing narratives from quantitative data, particularly data which have a temporal or longitudinal component. Data with narrative potential include large-scale prospective panel surveys (sometimes with links to census or other administrative data) which allow comparison over time, retrospective surveys which provide event histories and cohort studies which follow a group through time. Statistical analysis of these sources can provide detailed understanding of events and life courses which result in detailed descriptions of sequences and patterns. Narrative descriptions may weave between details of individual lives and the pattern of groups of lives, thus combining idiographic and nomothetic approaches. Elliott (2006) noted that such narratives more often focus on temporal patterns and changes than on the other common narrative purpose of making meaning.

Counting

Counting things reflects the 'numbered nature of phenomena' (Sandelowski 2001: 231) and is part of the descriptive process. Counting is a precursor to analysis (Morgan 1993) which recognises that data inherently combine quantitative and qualitative features (Coxon 2005). Use of counts communicates more effectively and reliably than does use of vague terms to indicate more or less frequent occurrence of some feature in the text (Miles and Huberman 1994; Sandelowski 2001). Counts can be viewed as reflecting the importance of various emergent themes (Onwuegbuzie and Teddlie 2003), although it can be argued that frequency and importance are not necessarily synonymous. Counting summarises patterns in data, allowing interrelationships to be more easily identified (Morgan 1993). It helps to maintain analytical integrity (as a counter to biased impressions), and can be used in verifying a hypothesis (Miles and Huberman 1994).

Counting themes, or instances of a category in a qualitative database, constitutes a very simple form of conversion of data from textual to numerical form. Indeed, for the majority of studies that develop quantitative reports from qualitative data, the quantitative data generated are just descriptive statistics reporting numbers of themes or categories found (Niglas 2004). Additionally, when subgroups are compared the resulting analyses provide not only an assessment of the qualitative differences in the coded text between the groups, but also a count of the number of members in each group coded for that concept. Verbatim transcripts of 158 initial genetic counselling sessions in a familial breast cancer clinic were coded by Butow and Lobb (2004) according to guidelines for best practice. The percentage of sessions in which each of a range of issues were discussed were reported, these tabulations showing that clinicians handled the clinical side of the sessions quite thoroughly, but were less effective in facilitating communication and emotional concerns. A count of lines of text without significant interruption showed that counsellors frequently spoke in long blocks when discussing the role of genes and chromosomes in breast cancer, and a count of the number of words spoken by each participant established that the clinician spoke approximately twice as much as the patient, overall.

Seale (2001) used counting in a slightly different way to investigate the use of 'struggle' language and sporting metaphors in media stories about people with cancer. Using Concordance, a word counting programme, he created a profile of words used in 358 texts depicting a person with cancer, out of which linguistic terms associated with military, sports and other metaphors were identified. Drawing on this sensitisation to language he then used NVivo to code and review the different ways in which struggle language was applied in the articles, with and without sporting connotations, in reports of people experiencing different types of cancer and in differing situations. Subsets of the text were further analysed with Concordance to provide a quantification of terms used in those different situations. This combination of iterative counting with discourse analysis enabled Seale (2001) to dispute previous theory and argue that the language used to describe peoples' experience with cancer was more sporting than militaristic in orientation. In a further analysis of messages from two popular media sites about decision making regarding treatment for breast and prostate cancers, Seale (2005) again used counts in combination with interpretive analysis of discourse to identify differences in the factors which are taken into consideration by men and women.

Whether one should use counts of the number of participants who mention something or the overall frequency with which something is mentioned depends on the context in which counts are being obtained and used and the possible meanings of a zero (0) count in that context. Similarly, the specificity of what is being counted impacts on meaning and use of counts, for example, whether it includes any reference to occupational stress as an issue, or just negative experiences of occupational stress (Bazeley 2003). Other problems which can occur when counting on the basis of qualitative coding relate to the use of percentages for small samples, relying on numbers to tell the whole story, and

not providing sufficient context to allow the reader to properly interpret the numbers (Sandelowski 2001).

Quantitising qualitative data

Transformation of data from verbal responses to numeric codes might
take place at any of a number of points during the research process,
including 1) during data collection by field staff, 2) categorising open-
ended responses in preparation for analysis, 3) conversion of qualitative codes to variable data during analysis, and 4) transformation after
analysis when results are being synthesised (Louis 1982). Such data
transformations are distinct from counting instances, and are usually
referred to as quantitising data (Tashakkori and Teddlie 1998). Usually,
decisions about how to use qualitative data quantitatively are made
before data are collected, '[h]owever, researchers who collect qualitative materials often develop schemes for quantifying their narrative
materials after the data have been gathered' (Polit and Hungler 1991:
499). Indeed, Louis (cited in Caracelli and Greene 1993) found she had
a large amount of rich and diverse data from multiple sites in a major
educational evaluation study, but that a complete dataset was available
for barely one-fifth of sites. She therefore created, at that point, a coding
form which could be applied across all sites in order to generate comparable data on 240 relevant holistic and specific variables.

Quantitisation is not always simply a matter of 0/1 transformation,
to indicate presence or absence of a code. In analysing comparable
simulated home visits to clients by 15 health visitors, Bryans (2004)
dealt with 'considerable' variations in the length of discussion of
various issues by weighting the coded excerpts 1–3 (representing variation from single statements to lengthy exchanges), making it possible
for her 'to identify dominant and recurring issues within the simulated
visits' (p. 627). In designing the software MaxQDA, Kuckartz (1995)
created a system in which the researcher can weight the code assigned
to a passage on a scale of 1–100, to record its significance in the context.
He recommends doing this on a second pass through the data, once
familiarity with the whole has been gained. Data might be quantified
in order to facilitate merging and comparison of different data sources
(Caracelli and Greene 1993; Happ et al. 2006; Creswell and Plano Clark
2007), or, with or without the addition of other quantitative data, to
allow exploratory, predictive or confirmatory statistical analyses.
'Methodologically speaking the aim must be to identify patterns in
social regularities and at the same time to understand them in the sense
of controlled *Fremdverstehen* (understanding the other)' (Kuckartz
1995: 158). Quantitising data is not an end in itself, but 'a means of

making available techniques which add power and sensitivity to individual judgment when one attempts to detect and describe patterning in a set of observations' (Weinstein and Tamur 1978: 140).

Quantitising to merge and compare

Traditionally those undertaking surveys which include open-ended questions have first categorised responses to those questions and then used that data in combination with other numerical or categorical responses in subsequent analysis, a procedure used, for example, by Bunn et al. (2006). Today, a variety of software programmes are available, including Wordstat and Statistical Packages for the Social Sciences (SPSS) text analysis software, which will more or less automatically categorise text responses so that they can be used in combination with other quantitative variables for further analysis. This approach might be considered to support mixed methods studies in that it generates quantitative variables from qualitative text, and allows for their combination with other quantitative data. If, however, no further reference is made to the detail of the qualitative material after conversion, they bear more resemblance to a purely quantitative analysis. Indeed, what is special about maintaining a mixed methods focus is that connection with the original text for interpretive purposes is retained, so that it remains possible to glean additional meaning from the statistical analysis, or to refer back and check the meaning or appropriateness of the variables that have been created.

Conversion to facilitate combination is a much broader practice than simply combining open and closed responses to a survey. Happ et al. (2006) recommend conversion and combination to reveal additional patterns and interpretations once data have been analysed within method. For example, they describe categorising a large amount of observational data to combine with physiological measures on weaning lung transplant patients from ventilators. They organised their data on an event-by-event basis with several entries for each person over time. The data were then able to be analysed to produce statistical trends and visual displays.

From interpretive phenomenological case studies of bi-monthly narratives from 60 male to male caregivers, provided over 2 years, Wrubel et al. (2001) distinguished and described three tacit definitions of caregiving. They then classified each caregiver as expressing either engagement, conflict or distance, and related that classification to scores indicating mood states, dyadic adjustment, interest in learning about how to care and involvement in health care decisions using matched t-tests and analyses of variance. Thus, a categorisation of participants based on narrative data facilitated statistical analyses linking those data to scaled scores on a case-by-case basis.

Innovative methods were used by Hume et al. (2005) to explore the relationship between children's environmental awareness and their level of physical activity. These researchers used children's maps of their home and neighbourhood as a way of identifying their perceptions of what environmental factors were important to them. The information in the maps was analysed qualitatively for descriptive themes. The six themes identified were then quantified in terms of the frequency with which particular objects and locations were included, to create 11 variables. Each child's level of physical activity was also measured using an accelerometer. While the results of the independent t-tests and bivariate linear regression analyses investigating the associations between each environmental variable and time spent in different intensities of physical activity for boys and girls were generally inconclusive, the methodology used was of interest and has potential for other settings.

Quantitising for exploration, prediction and explanation

Qualitative coding from free-flowing text is generally transformed into statistical data as a case-by-variable matrix, that is, a tabulation of either the presence or absence, or the frequency of occurrence of each code (in columns) for each case (in rows). Qualitative data analysis software (such as NVivo, MaxQDA, or QDA Miner) is particularly beneficial in being able to assist with this process, with QDA Miner providing inbuilt statistical processing and NVivo providing charting facilities. For each, case-based data can be exported to Excel or as a delimited text file, and then imported to any statistical program for further analysis using standard bivariate and multivariate comparative or regression-based techniques.

Coded interview data, supplemented by Kolb's learning styles inventory, were used by Carnwell (2000) to identify three types of distance learners, which they named systematic waders, speedy-focusers and global dippers, among a sample of nurses engaging in further study. The interviews were also coded for other learning issues that were then considered in association with the learning styles so as to predict participants' learning support needs. Initial conclusions were drawn from the qualitative analysis, but then the coding information was transferred to SPSS for statistical analysis. Logistic regression was used to build models of significant relationships between variables for each type of learner, some supporting and others refuting the tentative models developed from the qualitative analysis. Global dippers, for example, engaged in minimalist learning and so had particular need for practical support and a higher level of guidance through well structured course materials if they were to become successful students.

There are multiple strategies one might employ for transforming qualitative data in such a way as to allow exploratory or explanatory statistical analyses. These strategies hinge on either identifying and counting key words in the texts, or on translating coding information from qualitative to quantitative form. Cluster analysis, multidimensional scaling (MDS), correspondence analysis and factor analysis are some of the exploratory techniques that have been applied to the resulting data matrices to generate metathemes, core dimensions or comparative analyses (Ryan and Bernard 2000, 2003). Data from lists, paired comparisons or pile sorts of extracted themes can be used in a similar way; for example, by applying MDS to identify dimensions from having a number of people do similarity sorts of segments of text or short data items. Where data can be sorted for different groups then comparative techniques such as discriminant function analysis might also be employed. Software may be used to generate the kinds of data matrices needed for MDS and other exploratory statistical techniques, based on intersections or co-occurrences of coding derived from either freeflowing or structured textual or visual data.

Concept mapping, where participants develop a series of statements about the topic of interest, and then group and rate a refined list of these for importance and feasibility, has been used to provide a basis for planning or evaluation in a number of health and social contexts, for example, in the Healthy Hawaii Initiative (Kane and Trochim 2007). Cluster analysis and MDS were applied to the data generated by the participants to produce visual maps of the key areas that need to be developed or evaluated, and plots of the relative importance and feasibility of working in each of those areas. These results were then fed back to the participants, in the form of visual displays, for discussion, further development and as input to strategic planning.

Data blending to create new variables

New or consolidated variables or datasets might be constructed from a combination of qualitative and quantitative sources for use in further analyses, most often with an initiation purpose or effect. Caracelli and Greene (1993) provide two examples. In one, a quantitative variable of principal support derived from a blend of information from teacher surveys and principal interviews predicted implementation of a new programme. In another, 'weaving together' of quantitative and qualitative datasets regarding a freshman skills programme prompted new questions and construction of a new, critical variable for student immersion which was found to impact on programme outcomes.

This strategy was used by Kemp (1999) when she found ambivalence in the spinal injured population about whether they would access services they had most complained about not having, even if they became available. Qualitative coding regarding attitude to use of services was combined with a quantitative variable reflecting current use of services to create a new composite variable which was used for further quantitative analyses, and then imported back into the qualitative database for further comparative textual analyses. While the former pointed to a perception of arbitrariness in distribution of community services, the latter revealed that service provision was, in fact, not so arbitrary, but rather, that services were allocated on the proviso that persons with spinal injuries adopt life plans which met the expectations of service providers, that is, to be different rather than ordinary.

Issues in transforming qualitative coding

Conversion of coding for statistical analysis raises a number of issues to be addressed by the researcher, in addition to those raised already in relation to counting:

- Statistical procedures, particularly those offering prediction of explanation, are often based on an assumption of normally distributed probabilistic random sampling, with associated requirements about adequacy of sample size. Such requirements are rarely met by samples from which qualitative data are drawn.
- Those using matrix data generated from qualitative coding need to be aware of the basis on which the matrix was created. For example, comparative tables are most often more akin to multiple response data than to a cross-tabulation suitable for chi-squared analysis of differences as the categories being compared across groups are rarely mutually exclusive. Matrices derived from co-occurrences of different codes in qualitative data generally provide counts of the number of instances or cases in which those co-occurrences occur, and can be regarded as similarity matrices which are then usually suitable for MDS. With these, care needs to be exercised in specifying how the counts are constructed so that overcounting does not occur because the co-occurrence in some instances involved two passages and in others only one. The joining strategy for hierarchical cluster analysis is another situation where decisions are impacted by the source and derivation of the data being used.
- The specificity of the codes used in different approaches has implications for transforming data. Variable codes, derived from quantitative sources, have a representational rather than instru-

mental focus, and typically coding is to strictly defined values. Theme coding of qualitative sources, in contrast, 'seeks a holistic understanding . . . gives preference to relevance and completeness at the cost of precision and selectivity' (Sivesind 1999: 365). Where qualitative theme coding of this type is quantitised, it may lack sufficient specificity to be useful. For example, if the act of a judge questioning the character of a witness is coded without identifying the conclusion reached, further coding of the original data into more specific categories may be required before the data are exported in variable form.

Further analytical strategies

In addition to the strategies already outlined, there are three broad groups of strategies which have been recognised by nurse researchers as being useful. These include iterative analysis; analysis of extreme, deviant, contrasting or negative cases; and visual display techniques. Other techniques which are yet to make a significant impact on nursing and health research, but which could well have value as a bridge between quantitative and qualitative approaches, include use of fuzzy sets and qualitative comparative analysis (Ragin 1987, 1995, 2000); Q-methodology (Brown 2006); the use of repertory grids (Kelly 1955, Rocco et al. 2003); and social network analysis (Scott 2000).

Iterative analysis

Iterative working between approaches often takes development or expansion a step further. Iteration involves taking what is learned in one stage of a project into a further stage to inform that data collection or analysis, and then on again for refinement or development through one or more subsequent iterations. Alternatively, it may be linked with typology development, where a typology developed from one approach is applied to data from another (Caracelli and Greene 1993).

Ahern (2002) used exploratory factor analysis to validate phenomenologically derived themes derived from interviews with parents whose child had developmental coordination disorder. Categories identified in the texts were clustered into themes, validated by experts, and pilot tested to develop an instrument which could then be used to assess the generalisability of the experiences reported by parents. Issues identified through the reclustering of items in the factor analysis, including identification of new themes, were taken back to the phenomenological data for further exploration and analysis.

Extreme, deviant, contrasting or negative case analyses

One of the interesting differences about the way those from differing analytical traditions deal with their data is their approach to extreme or deviant cases. In statistical analyses, particularly those based on linear regression models, it is often necessary to remove 'outlier' cases as they have a disproportionate skewing effect on the results of the analysis (Tabachnick and Fidell 1996). In contrast, these cases are often regarded as being of particular interest in qualitative approaches, as the goal for any explanation derived from the data is that it can account for all cases (Miles and Huberman 1994; Maxwell 2005). In addition, these cases often bring to light critical new considerations for the analysis. Fielding and Fielding (1986) referred to Cressey's (1953) study of embezzlers in which he had to keep revising his conclusions after considering negative cases. In so doing he came up with four necessary conditions for embezzlement to occur which explained 100% of cases. They note that in qualitative analysis 'there is no random error variance. All exceptions are eliminated by revising hypotheses until all the data fit' (Fielding and Fielding 1986: 89).

Extreme, deviant or negative cases identified from analysis of one data type can be pursued using the other, perhaps with the results of that analysis then being fed back as a modification to the original analysis (Caracelli and Greene 1993). These might be cases identified through comparative text analysis as not fitting a pattern, those identified as having high residuals in a regression, or those scoring in the top and bottom deciles of a sample on a quantitative measure. For example, in examining conceptions of abuse in relation to experience of domestic violence, West and Tulloch (2001) selected as a sample for interview those whose self-definition was not correctly predicted by a discriminant function analysis of survey data, with each interview being informed by responses from the survey.

Visual display techniques

The case for visual display of data was argued very strongly by Miles and Huberman (1994) who made extensive use of matrix displays for pattern analysis along with other visual techniques, including use of flow charts and positioning cases on orthogonal axes. Metamatrices, scatterplots, bar graphs, clustered (comparative) bar graphs and modified stem and leaf plots using case numbers against qualitative themes were strategies suggested by Happ et al. (2006) for visually displaying combinations of qualitative and quantitative data. To display data, one must understand the data: both the task of constructing a display and viewing a finished display stimulate and clarify interpretation of data.

When quantitised coding is explored statistically, the resulting multidimensional plots (from MDS or correspondence analysis) or dendrograms (from cluster analysis) assist interpretation of the data. Mapping the clustering of important neighbourhood domains for women experiencing intimate partner violence revealed, for O'Campo et al. (2005), the pathways through which the local neighbourhood potentially influenced the perpetration, severity and cessation of intimate partner violence. Kane and Trochim (2007) provided examples of a range of visual displays developed through applying a combination of cluster analysis and MDS to paired and rated statements, in the context of concept mapping for health and social planning and evaluation. Ryan and Bernard (2000) also provided multiple examples of visual displays created through MDS and similar techniques, derived from combinations of qualitative and quantitative data.

The role of interpretation in the construction of knowledge

Fielding and Fielding (1986) are not alone in having noted the interpretive quality of all data, yet researchers typically place great reliance on the probability value which is generated from inferential testing in statistical analysis. This value, however, is highly dependent on sample size (as well as sample variance). Test with a large enough sample and you are very likely to find that a very small difference will become 'significant'. But is that difference meaningful? And might not differences which are not statistically significant still have meaning? The first question is well illustrated by DeVito Dabbs et al. (2004) where they note that a difference which was statistically significant should be ignored as it was not clinically significant. The second can be illustrated by the example of a situation, often encountered in analysing survey data, where age differences recorded in decades are not significant, but an examination of the data reveals that those who are over 60 are indeed quite different from all other groups, it is just that their difference was hidden by the structure of the data. The point is:

> From data in the form of numbers, one makes inferences in the same way as with data in the form of words, not by virtue of probabilistic algorithms. Statistics are not privileged. Inference is not mechanised. With this way of viewing knowledge, 'mixed' methods may even be a misnomer, as both surveys and participant observation yield equivalent data. Inferences are based on

the inquirer's coordinating multiple lines of evidence to gain an overall understanding of the phenomenon . . . Yet, because the inquirer is the instrument, all information flows through a single perspective . . . the standard of a valid account rests on establishing coherence across multiple lines of evidence and argument (Smith 1997: 77).

Coyle and Williams (2000) recommend 'extending the concept of reflexivity (used in qualitative research) to the quantitative components of mixed method studies. This would aid conceptual clarity by making explicit the social, cultural and political construction of knowledge, and would also encourage researchers to reflect upon the ethical and political consequences of their research' (p. 1235).

The essential nature of analysis, as the ability to gather, order, evaluate and interpret evidence, overrides 'qualitative' and 'quantitative' distinctions in the nature of the evidence or the methods for working with it. With their consequent potential to more fully exploit the multiple data sources available to them, nurse and health science researchers who understand this can move beyond the limitations of current research practice in their quest to construct new knowledge and improve professional practice.

References

Ahern K. (2002) Developmental coordination disorder: validation of a qualitative analysis using statistical factor analysis. *International Journal of Qualitative Methods*, **1**(3), Article 5. Accessed 6 October 2004 from http://www.ualberta.ca/~ijqm.

Andrew S. and Halcomb E.J. (2006) Mixed methods research is an effective method of enquiry for working with families and communities. *Contemporary Nurse*, **23**(2), 145–153.

Barbour R.S. (1998) Mixing qualitative methods: quality assurance or qualitative quagmire? *Qualitative Health Research*, **8**(3), 352–361.

Bazeley P. (2003) Computerized data analysis for mixed methods research. In Tashakkori A. and Teddlie C. (eds.) *Handbook of Mixed Methods in Social and Behavioral Research*, pp. 385–422. Thousand Oaks, CA: Sage.

Bazeley P. (2004) Issues in mixing qualitative and quantitative approaches to research. In Buber R., Gadner J. and Richards L. (eds.) *Applying Qualitative Methods to Marketing Management Research*, pp. 141–156. Basingstoke, UK: Palgrave Macmillan.

Bazeley P. (2006) The contribution of computer software to integrating qualitative and quantitative data and analyses. *Research in the Schools*, **13**(1), 63–73.

Bazeley P. (2007) *Qualitative Data Analysis with NVivo*. London: Sage.

Beringer A.J., Fletcher M.E. and Taket A.R. (2006) Rules and resources: a structuration approach to understanding the coordination of children's inpatient health care. *Journal of Advanced Nursing*, **56**(3), 325–335.

Brewer J. and Hunter A. (2006) *Foundations of Multimethod Research: Synthesizing Styles*. Thousand Oaks, CA: Sage.

Brown S.R. (2006) A match made in heaven: a marginalized methodology for studying the marginalized. *Quality and Quantity*, **40**(3), 361–382.

Bryans A.N. (2004) Examining health visiting expertise: combining simulation, interview and observation. *Journal of Advanced Nursing*, **47**(6), 623–630.

Bryman A. (2006) Integrating quantitative and qualitative research: how is it done? *Qualitative Research*, **6**(1), 97–113.

Bryman A. (2007) Barriers to integrating quantitative and qualitative research. *Journal of Mixed Methods Research*, **1**(1), 8–22.

Bunn H., Lange I., Urrutia M., Campos M.S., Campos S., Jaimovich S. et al. (2006) Health preferences and decision-making needs of disadvantaged women. *Journal of Advanced Nursing*, **56**(3), 247–260.

Butow P.N. and Lobb E.A. (2004) Analysing the process and content of genetic counseling in familial breast cancer consultations. *Journal of Genetic Counseling*, **13**(5), 403–424.

Caracelli V. and Greene J. (1993) Data analysis strategies for mixed-method evaluation designs. *Educational Evaluation and Policy Analysis*, **15**(2), 195–207.

Carey L.K., Nicholson B.C. and Fox R.A. (2002) Maternal factors related to parenting young children with congenital heart disease. *Journal of Pediatric Nursing: Nursing Care of Children and Families*, **17**(3), 174–183.

Carnwell R. (2000) Pedagogical implications of approaches to study in distance learning: developing models through qualitative and quantitative analysis. *Journal of Advanced Nursing*, **31**(5), 1018–1028.

Coxon A.P.M. (2005) Integrating qualitative and quantitative data: what does the user need? *Forum: Qualitative Social Research*, **6**(2), www.qualitative-research.net/index.php/fqs/article/view/463/991.

Coyle J. and Williams B. (2000) An exploration of the epistemological intricacies of using qualitative data to develop a quantitative measure of user views of health care. *Journal of Advanced Nursing*, **31**(5), 1235–1243.

Creswell J.W. (2003) *Research Design: Qualitative, Quantitative and Mixed Methods Approaches*. Thousand Oaks, CA: Sage.

Creswell J.W. and Plano Clark V.L. (2007) *Designing and Conducting Mixed Methods Research*. Thousand Oaks, CA: Sage.

DeVito Dabbs A., Hoffman L.A., Swigart V., Happ M.B., Iacono A.T. and Dauber J.H. (2004) Using conceptual triangulation to develop an integrated model of the symptom experience of acute rejection after lung transplantation. *Advances in Nursing Science*, **27**(2), 138–149.

Elliott J. (2005) *Using Narrative in Social Research: Qualitative and Quantitative Approaches*. London: Sage.

Erzberger C. and Kelle U. (2003) Making inferences in mixed methods: the rules of integration. In Tashakkori A. and Teddlie C. (eds.) *Handbook of Mixed Methods in Social and Behavioral Research*, pp. 457–488. Thousand Oaks, CA: Sage.

Fielding N.G. and Fielding J.L. (1986) *Linking Data: the Articulation of Qualitative and Quantitative Methods in Social Research* (Qualitative Research Methods Series No. 4). Beverly Hills, CA: Sage.

Flensner G. and Lindencrona C. (2002) The cooling-suit: case studies of its influence on fatigue among eight individuals with multiple sclerosis. *Journal of Advanced Nursing*, **37**(6), 541–550.

Ford R.T. (2006) *Nursing attitudes and therapeutic capacity: what are the implications for nursing care of patients who use illicit drugs?* Unpublished doctoral dissertation, Australian National University, Canberra.

Foster R.L. (1997) Addressing epistemologic and practical issues in multi-method research: a procedure for conceptual triangulation. *Advances in Nursing Science*, **20**(1), 1–12.

Ginsburg K.R., Howe C.J., Jawad A.F., Buzby M., Ayala J.M., Tuttle A. et al. (2005) Parents' perceptions of factors that affect successful diabetes management for their children. *Pediatrics*, **116**(5), 1095–1104.

Greene J C., Caracelli V.J. and Graham W.F. (1989) Toward a conceptual framework for mixed-method evaluation designs. *Educational Evaluation and Policy Analysis*, **11**(3), 255–274.

Happ M.B., DeVito Dabbs A., Tate J., Hricik A. and Erlen J. (2006) Exemplars of mixed methods data combination and analysis. *Nursing Research*, **55**(2, Supplement 1), S43–S49.

Harden A. and Thomas J. (2005) Methodological issues in combining diverse study types in systematic reviews. *International Journal of Social Research Methodology*, **8**(3), 257–271.

Hildebrandt E. and Kelber S.T. (2005) Perceptions of health and well-being among women in a work-based welfare program. *Public Health Nursing*, **22**(6), 506–514.

Hume C., Salmon J. and Ball K. (2005) Children's perceptions of their home and neighborhood environments, and their association with objectively measured physical activity: a qualitative and quantitative study. *Health Education Research*, **20**(1), 1–13.

Jick T.D. (1979) Mixing qualitative and quantitative methods: triangulation in action. *Administrative Science Quarterly*, **24**, 602–611.

Jones A. and Bugge C. (2006) Improving understanding and rigour through triangulation: an exemplar based on patient participation in interaction. *Journal of Advanced Nursing*, **55**(5), 612–621.

Kane M. and Trochim W. (2007) *Concept Mapping for Planning and Evaluation*. Thousand Oaks, CA: Sage.

Kanzaki H., Makimoto K., Takemura T. and Ashida N. (2004) Development of web-based qualitative and quantitative data collection systems: study on daily symptoms and coping strategies among Japanese rheumatoid arthritis patients. *Nursing and Health Sciences*, **6**(3), 229–236.

Kelly G. (1955) *The Psychology of Personal Constructs*. New York: Norton.

Kemp L.A. (1999) *Charting a parallel course: meeting the community service needs of persons with spinal injuries*. Unpublished doctoral dissertation, University of Western Sydney, Campbelltown, NSW.

Kinn S. and Curzio J. (2005) Integrating qualitative and quantitative research methods. *Journal of Research in Nursing*, **10**(3), 317–336.

Knafl K.A. and Ayres L. (1996) Managing large qualitative data sets in family research. *Journal of Family Nursing*, **2**(4), 350–364.

Kuckartz U. (1995) Case-oriented quantification. In Kelle U. (ed.) *Computer-aided Qualitative Data Analysis: Theory, Methods and Practice*, pp. 158–176. Thousand Oaks, CA: Sage.

Louis K.S. (1982) Multisite/multimethod studies. *American Behavioral Scientist*, **26**(1), 6–22.

Maliski S.L., Sarna L., Evangelista L. and Padilla G. (2003) The aftermath of lung cancer: balancing the good and bad. *Cancer Nursing*, **26**(3), 237–244.

Martin L., Farrell M., Lambrenos K. and Nayagam D. (2003) Living with the Ilizarov frame: adolescent perceptions. *Journal of Advanced Nursing*, **43**(5), 478–487.

Mathison S. (1988) Why triangulate? *Educational Researcher*, **17**(2), 13–17.

Maxwell J. (2005) *Qualitative Research Design*. Thousand Oaks, CA: Sage.

Maxwell J. and Loomis D. (2003) Mixed method design: an alternative approach. In Tashakkori A. and Teddlie C. (eds.) *Handbook of Mixed Methods in Social and Behavioral Research*, pp. 241–271. Thousand Oaks, CA: Sage.

McKeon C.M., Fogarty G.J. and Hegney D.G. (2006) Organizational factors: impact on administration violations in rural nursing. *Journal of Advanced Nursing*, **55**(1), 115–123.

Meetoo D. and Temple B. (2003) Issues in multi-method research: constructing self-care. *International Journal of Qualitative Methods*, 2, Article 1. Accessed 6 October 2004 from http://www.ualberta.ca/~iiqm/.

Miles M.B. and Huberman A.M. (1994) *Qualitative Data Analysis: an Expanded Sourcebook*. Thousand Oaks, CA: Sage.

Moran-Ellis J., Alexander V.D., Cronin A., Dickinson M., Fielding J., Sleney J. and Thomas H. (2006) Triangulation and integration: processes, claims and implications. *Qualitative Research*, **6**(1), 45–59.

Morgan D.L. (1993) Qualitative content analysis: a guide to paths not taken. *Qualitative Health Research*, **3**(1), 112–121.

Morgan D.L. (2007) Paradigms lost and pragmatism regained: methodological implications of combining qualitative and quantitative methods. *Journal of Mixed Methods Research*, **1**(1), 48–76.

Morse J.M. (2003) Principles of mixed methods and multimethod research design. In Tashakkori A. and Teddlie C. (eds.) *Handbook of Mixed Methods in Social and Behavioral Research*, pp. 189–208. Thousand Oaks, CA: Sage.

Nickel B., Berger M., Schmidt P. and Plies K. (1995) Qualitative sampling in a multi-method survey. *Quality and Quantity*, **29**, 223–240.

Niglas K. (2004) *The Combined Use of Qualitative and Quantitative Methods in Educational Research*. Tallin, Estonia: Tallinn Pedagogical University.

Niglas K. (2007) Review of: Microsoft Office Excel spreadsheet software. *Journal of Mixed Methods Research*, **1**(3), 297.

O'Campo P., Burke J., Peak G.L., McDonnell K.A. and Gielen A.C. (2005) Uncovering neighbourhood influences on intimate partner violence using concept mapping. *Journal of Epidemiology and Community Health*, **59**(7), 603–608.

O'Cathain A., Murphy E. and Nicholl J. (2007) Integration and publications as indicators of 'yield' from mixed methods studies. *Journal of Mixed Methods Research*, **1**(2), 147–163.

Ong B.N., Dunn K.M. and Croft P.R. (2006) 'Since you're asking . . .': free text commentaries in an epidemiological study of low back pain consulters in primary care. *Quality and Quantity*, **40**, 651–659.

Onwuegbuzie A.J. and Teddlie C. (2003) A framework for analyzing data in mixed methods research. In Tashakkori A. and Teddlie C. (eds.) *Handbook of Mixed Methods in Social and Behavioral Research*, pp. 351–384. Thousand Oaks, CA: Sage.

Patton M.Q. (1988) Paradigms and pragmatism. In Fetterman D.M. (ed.) *Qualitative Approaches to Evaluation in Education: the Silent Scientific Revolution*, pp. 116–137. New York: Praeger.

Polit D.F. and Hungler B.P. (1991) *Nursing Research: Principles and Methods*. Philadelphia: J.B. Lippincott.

Ragin C. (1987) *The Comparative Method: Moving Beyond Qualitative and Quantitative Strategies*. Berkeley, CA: University of California Press.

Ragin C.C. (1995) Using qualitative comparative analysis to study configurations. In Kelle U. (ed.) *Computer-aided Qualitative Data Analysis: Theory, Methods and Practice*, pp. 177–189. Thousand Oaks, CA: Sage.

Ragin C. (2000) *Fuzzy-set Social Science*. Chicago: University of Chicago Press.

Rocco T.S., Bliss L.A., Gallagher S., Perez-Prado A., Alacaci C., Dwyer E.S., Fine J.C. and Pappamihiel N.E. (2003) The pragmatic and dialectical lenses: two views of mixed methods use in education. In Tashakkori A. and Teddlie C. (eds.) *Handbook of Mixed Methods in Social and Behavioral Research*, pp. 595–615. Thousand Oaks, CA: Sage.

Ryan G.W. and Bernard H.R. (2000) Data management and analysis methods. In Denzin N. and Lincoln Y. (eds.) *Handbook of Qualitative Research*, 2nd edition, pp. 769–802. Thousand Oaks: Sage.

Ryan G.W. and Bernard H.R. (2003) Techniques to identify themes. *Field Methods*, **15**(1), 85–109.

Sale J.E.M., Lohfield L. and Brazil K. (2002) Revisiting the quantitative–qualitative debate: implications for mixed-methods research. *Quality and Quantity*, **36**, 43–53.

Sandelowski M. (1995) On the aesthetics of qualitative research. *IMAGE: Journal of Nursing Scholarship*, **27**, 205–209.

Sandelowski M. (2000) Combining qualitative and quantitative sampling, data collection, and analysis techniques in mixed-method studies. *Research in Nursing and Health*, **23**(3), 246–255.

Sandelowski M. (2001) Real qualitative researchers do not count: the use of numbers in qualitative research. *Research in Nursing and Health*, **24**(3), 230–240.

Sandelowski M., Voils C.I. and Barroso J. (2006) Defining and designing mixed research synthesis studies. *Research in the Schools*, **13**(1), 29–40.

Schrijnemaekers V.J.J., van Rossum E., van Heusden M.J.T. and Widdershoven G.A.M. (2002) Compliance in a randomized controlled trial: the implementation of emotion-orientated care in psycho-geriatric facilities. *Journal of Advanced Nursing*, **39**(2), 182–189.

Scott J. (2000) *Social Network Analysis: a Handbook*. London: Sage.

Seale C.F. (2001) Sporting cancer: struggle language in news reports of people with cancer. *Sociology of Health and Illness*, **23**(3), 308–329.

Seale C. (2005) Portrayals of treatment decision-making on popular breast and prostate cancer web sites. *European Journal of Cancer Care*, **14**(2), 171–174.

Simons L. (2007) Moving from collision to integration. *Journal of Research in Nursing*, **12**(1), 73–83.

Sivesind K. (1999) Structured, qualitative comparison: between singularity and single-dimensionality. *Quality and Quantity*, **33**, 361–380.

Smith M.L. (1997) Mixing and matching: methods and models. In Greene J.C. and Caracelli V.J. (eds.) *Advances in Mixed-method Evaluation: The Challenges and Benefits of Integrating Diverse Paradigms*, pp. 73–86. San Francisco: Jossey-Bass.

Tabachnick B.G. and Fidell L.S. (1996) *Using Multivariate Statistics*. New York: Harper Collins.

Tashakkori A. and Teddlie C. (1998) *Mixed Methodology: Combining Qualitative and Quantitative Approaches*. Thousand Oaks, CA: Sage.

Tolson D., Smith M. and Knight P. (1999) An investigation of the components of best nursing practice in the care of acutely ill hospitalized older patients with coincidental dementia: a multi-method design. *Journal of Advanced Nursing*, **30**(5), 1127–1136.

Weinstein E.A. and Tamur J.M. (1978) Meanings, purposes, and structural resources in social interaction. In Manis J.G. and Meltzer B.N. (eds.) *Symbolic Interaction*, 3rd edition, pp. 138–140. Boston: Allyn and Bacon.

Wendler M.C. (2001) Triangulation using a meta-matrix. *Journal of Advanced Nursing*, **35**(4), 521–525.

West E. and Tulloch M. (2001) Qualitising quantitative data: should we do it, and if so, how? Paper presented at *Annual Conference of the Australian Association for Social Research* 19 May, Wollongong, NSW.

Wrubel J., Richards T.A., Folkman S. and Acree M.C. (2001) Tacit definitions of informal caregiving. *Journal of Advanced Nursing*, **33**(2), 175–181.

Yin R.K. (2006) Mixed methods research: are the methods genuinely integrated or merely parallel? *Research in the Schools*, **13**(1), 41–47.

Acknowledgement

Early work on this chapter was completed while I was 2006 Visiting International Fellow at the Institute of Social Research, University of Surrey.

From Rigour to Trustworthiness: Validating Mixed Methods

Lynne S. Giddings and Barbara M. Grant

Learning objectives

The aim of this chapter is to provide the reader with an understanding of the complexity involved in validating mixed methods research. The chapter will explore how concepts such as rigour, reliability, trustworthiness and validity can be applied by those undertaking mixed methods research.

After reading this chapter, you will have the knowledge to:

a) Explain the importance and purpose of ensuring validation within mixed methods research.
b) Understand the shift in the meaning of validation between quantitative rigour, which includes notions like reliability and validity, and qualitative trustworthiness, with notions like credibility and fittingness.
c) Differentiate the numerous approaches to validation in mixed methods within the context of different research paradigms.

Introduction

To ensure the quality of mixed methods research, explicit criteria by which both the quantitative and qualitative components of the investigation can be validated are required. Validation in mixed methods, however, requires more than simply applying the traditional scientific principles of rigour. The 'mix' in mixed methods can come from within and across a variety of research paradigms (see Chapter 2). Given the variety of ways in which the 'mix' of qualitative and quantitative can be achieved, there are various means of establishing validation. In our experience, health and social science students undertaking research for the first time often struggle with the inevitable complexities of validating their research designs. This complexity is only compounded when using a mixed methods approach.

If there is incongruence between the design and the validation principles applied, a researcher may find that they cannot support their conclusions, nor convincingly answer their research question. It is important, therefore, that when designing and undertaking a mixed methods study, the strategies used to ensure the overall validity of the work are made explicit. In this chapter we use a particular paradigm framework (Grant and Giddings 2002) to address validation in diverse research contexts. We conclude the chapter by discussing issues that can arise when using a mixed methods approach that crosses research paradigms.

Paradigm framework

As described in Grant and Giddings (2002), there are four main health and social science research paradigms, the positivist/postpositivist paradigm which has been traditionally labelled 'quantitative research', and the interpretivist/constructivist, radical/critical and poststructural/postmodern paradigms which are often clumped together as 'qualitative research' (Box 7.1). A researcher's paradigm reflects their beliefs about what reality is (ontology), what counts as knowledge (epistemology), how we gain knowledge (methodology) and the values we hold (axiology). Taken together, paradigmatic assumptions and

---

Box 7.1 Point to ponder

Health and social science research can generally be placed within one of four research paradigms: positivism/postpositivism, interpretivism/constructivism, critical/radical, poststructural/postmodern. When qualitative and quantitative methods are mixed within a study they are usually situated within one worldview or paradigm. Validation strategies differ depending on which paradigm the study is positioned within.

beliefs not only guide the choice of methodology and methods and the nature of the researcher–researched relationship, but also the ways in which the validity of the research is assessed and ensured. Before discussing the paradigms and their associated forms of validation, we distinguish the meanings of the often confused terms 'methodology' and 'methods' as this distinction is important for our understanding of validation.

'Methodology' and 'methods'

As has been discussed in Chapter 1, 'methodology' is an abstract term that refers to the theoretical assumptions and principles that underpin a particular research approach. Methodology is a *thinking tool* that guides how a researcher frames the research question and decides on what processes and methods to use, including how to establish the validation of a study (Giddings and Grant 2007). Methods, in contrast, are much more concrete and practical – they are the *doing tools* for collecting and analysing data, and for establishing validity. The methods a researcher chooses to ensure research validation need to fit with their methodology which in turn must be congruent with the overall purpose of the study. See Box 7.2.

Box 7.2 Research in action

In their mixed methods evaluation of a model of nursing care for older patients, Glasson et al. (2006) used the methodology of action research. The methods used to collect data included interviews, questionnaires, validated instruments and the researchers' field notes.

Shifting meanings of rigour

Historically, the idea of rigour has dominated discussions of ensuring research quality. The terms reliability and validity have been synonymous with rigour within positivist scientific research and underpin a study's claim to generalisability (Patton 2002). The application of these terms to mixed methods research seemed quite logical, particularly as the use of both qualitative and quantitative methods of data collection in a single study has been viewed as a way to ensure rigour.

Indeed, until recently, positivist assumptions in their various forms have underpinned the majority of mixed methods designs used in nursing research (Giddings and Williams 2006). Giddings and Williams' (2006) review of mixed methods research published in nursing journals between 1998 and 2005 found that the methods mixed were often descriptive, with the qualitative component for the most part viewed as complementary but subordinate to the quantitative data collection.

In the late 1980s and into the 1990s, with the increasing influence of postpositivist values on scientific research, there was a more general acceptance of non-positivist qualitative research approaches (Tashakkori and Teddlie 2003). This influence, combined with funding bodies' demands for a more comprehensive picture of various health problems and issues, led to the use of a variety of qualitative methodologies from different paradigmatic positions within mixed methods studies (e.g.: phenomenology, grounded theory, feminist research) (Giddings 2006). Combining qualitative and quantitative approaches had already made apparent the limitations of the scientific understanding of rigour and the assumption of generalisability but, with the inclusion of interpretive, critical and poststructural qualitative methodologies in mixed methods studies, the concept of rigour needed to be expanded. Hence our choice of the term 'validation' rather than rigour as the umbrella concept for processes which ensure quality in research.

The processes for ensuring research validation must shift and change depending on which research paradigm is dominant within the mixed methods design (refer to Chapter 3). In a postpositivist mixed methods study, where both the quantitative and qualitative methods are descriptive (e.g. a questionnaire with descriptive statistical analysis and semi-structured interviews with quasi-statistical or descriptive content analysis), the processes of reliability, validity and generalisability are applied. If the qualitative analysis moves from categorical content analysis into a more abstracted mode of interpretation, such as thematic content analysis, then extra validation strategies of 'trustworthiness' are also applied; that is, processes must be adopted to ensure that the interpretation of the researcher and the conclusions made are credible and trustworthy (Lincoln and Guba 1985). Although the idea of trustworthiness emerges in postpositivist research that uses this kind of qualitative data analysis, the meanings of trustworthiness, and the processes used to enact it, alter across the various qualitative research paradigms. In mixed methods studies that use a non-positivist qualitative methodology, there is a critical shift from research claims that depend on quantitative data to those that depend on qualitative data. In other words, there is a shift from the use of objective tools and measurement, and the norms of reliability, validity and generalisability.

Instead the trustworthiness of the researcher is emphasised, the norms of reliability and validity shift in meaning, and the idea of transferability replaces generalisability.

The differences between paradigms mean there is no one way or specific set of standards to ensure validation in mixed methods research. Rather there is a need to understand what is being mixed, so as to decide whether or not more than one set of validation strategies should be applied. Using mixed methods requires being 'vigorously self-aware' (Lather 1986: 66) of paradigmatic positioning and how this influences decisions concerning validation. Otherwise there is a tendency to be drawn back into the positivist desire for certainty and the defensive application of the traditional standards of rigour. What is important for all validation strategies is that they are congruent with the theoretical assumptions underpinning a study's dominant paradigm.

Positivist/postpositivist validation strategies

Within the positivist/postpositivist paradigm, social reality is viewed as relatively stable and based on pre-existing patterns or order (Grant and Giddings 2002). Research from within this paradigm aims to gain knowledge about the world in order to explain, predict or control events (Polit and Beck 2006). Such 'facts' or 'evidence' can be found through using quantitative and qualitative methods which, when mixed, create a specific body of knowledge about an event or an issue. A mixed methods study from this paradigm follows a detailed protocol outlining all the steps involved in the quantitative and qualitative methods and is developed prior to the beginning of data collection and analysis.

Research validation assumes the scientific standards of rigour. Validation within this paradigm has been usefully defined as 'the ability of the researcher to draw meaningful and accurate conclusions from all of the data in the study' (Creswell and Plano Clark 2007: 146). Whether the method is quantitative or qualitative, scientifically rigorous strategies are applied to ensure that the methods of data collection and analysis are reliable and valid. Tashakkori and Teddlie (2003) refer to this process as ensuring 'inference quality' – the accuracy with which researchers draw inductive and deductive conclusions from a study. This process takes time but, once internal consistency and feasibility are established, and an appropriate population accessed, the study is completed relatively quickly.

To enable an understanding of the rigour procedures for positivist/postpositivist mixed methods studies, we will treat the quantitative and qualitative rigour strategies separately. However, in the reality of conducting this research, both strategies work together to provide confidence in the overall integrity of a study.

Rigour in the quantitative component

There are numerous designs within the non-experimental and experimental research categories that can be used in mixed methods research. Therefore, the following discussion will deal with general, rather than specific, validation strategies. What needs to be remembered is that the rigour processes used in non-experimental descriptive methods, including correlational designs, can also be applied in experimental research. For example, a questionnaire may be used in a quality-of-life study of people with chronic pain. Used in a non-experimental study, the questionnaire may describe the characteristics of chronic pain. However, in an experimental study, the same questionnaire may be used as an outcome measure to facilitate the researcher making comparisons over time to see if an intervention (independent variable) has made a difference in relation to a measured outcome (dependent variable). The strategies that are applied to ensure that the questionnaire is reliable and valid are the same in both studies.

In quantitative research to establish the validity of a study means that a researcher can draw meaningful inferences from the results gained from a sample (n) to a population (N). In other words, the findings are generalisable. To achieve this, the way the tools or instruments are constructed and how they are used must be reliable and valid (*measurement validity*), and the research study is designed in such a way that it does what is intended (*design validity*).

Measurement validity

The goal of measurement validity is to ensure that instruments, such as questionnaires and audit tools, consistently and reliably measure something. *Reliability* means that scores attained by a respondent on a questionnaire, for example, are consistent and stable over time. This process involves external validation processes such as statistical procedures of internal consistency (reliability coefficient) and instrument test–retest comparisons. The *validity* of the instrument is also established through face validity. *Face validity* of a questionnaire, for example, is when a researcher concludes that on the face of it the questions reflect and are relevant to the topic being explored. *Content validity* gives more evidence that questionnaire items can be trusted as representative of the content they were intended to measure. The evidence is provided by known experts in the area of interest who judge the items against certain criteria and conclude and come to a consensus, that yes they do relate and are relevant to the issue being studied.

Measurement validity is also related to a researcher being confident that the scores achieved by respondents have relevance. This can be ascertained by a process of *criterion-related validity*, where the scores gained on the instrument are able to relate to some external standard or that similar scores are produced on an instrument that pertains to measure the same thing. In other words, the results obtained when using a study's questionnaire correlate with the other instrument's results. A more complex, but more convincing approach, is establishing the *construct validity* of an instrument – what construct (variable) is the instrument actually measuring? The *known-groups technique* is one strategy commonly used; a prediction is made from an assumption that certain groups will differ on a particular behaviour or response. So, for example, one might assume that women having their first baby might have more anxiety than women having their second or third. If there is no difference and you have a large number of participants in your sample, then one might question the construct validity of the instrument. A more convincing strategy is factor analysis which involves a statistical procedure. On a questionnaire, clusters are made of items that share common characteristics or underlying assumptions, so that the different groupings are distinguishable from one another.

Design validity

In experimental studies the study needs to be designed in such a way as to reduce the threats to *internal validity* and *external validity*. Internal validity means that the researcher can only draw cause-and-effect inferences from the sample (n) to the population (N) if various threats are accounted for in the design (such as selection bias, attrition of participants, ageing of the sample group and so on). External validity is the extent to which the results can be applied to other groups or situations other than the sample group, if various threats (extraneous variables) are controlled for (such as the Hawthorne effect and placebo effect). Such generalisability to other groups or settings is important as it gives evidence that a study design is able to do what it was intended to do.

Rigour in the qualitative component

In many mixed methods studies qualitative data is used to support the quantitative findings. Most commonly, a questionnaire or validated instruments/scales are followed by interviews so that examples can be given of the respondent's experience of a particular situation. In these designs, the qualitative findings complement or expand the understanding of the quantitative data. For example, in a study of appearance-related concerns of people with visible disfigurement, Rumsey et al. (2004) used cross-sectional survey design followed by semi-structured interviews to 'generate further quantitative and qualitative data about individual concerns, and satisfaction with the provision of care' (p. 443).

The second most common design is when a semi-structured interview is used to collect information which can guide the development of a questionnaire. These two designs involve descriptive qualitative methods. What needs to be determined for validity purposes is whether the account provided by the participants, as well as the interpretation given by the researcher, work together to produce accurate and credible findings that can be trusted. We argue that trustworthiness is related to the data collection and analysis processes rather than the trustworthiness or the interpretive ability of the researcher as in the interpretive/constructivist paradigm.

Validation strategies

Validation of postpositivist qualitative research relies upon using all or most of the following strategies. Our account here draws heavily on the work of Patton (2002) and Creswell and Plano Clark (2007).

The first strategy involves clear articulation of the *research question*. Clarification of this question is important as it guides the data collection and analysis process and is expected to be answered by the findings. Questions tend to focus on describing something, such as factors, characteristics or attributes.

The second strategy is *triangulation*, that is, the use of more than one method of data collection (e.g. interviews and observation) or sources of data (e.g. interviews with clients, family and nurses). This process is seen as a way of ensuring the validity of the findings through comprehensiveness and the convergence of patterns (internal agreement); one method is expected to compensate for the weakness of another.

By providing a clear account of the process of data collection and analysis, the researcher is able to establish *auditability*. A researcher needs to show, for example, how a coding system was used to establish categories and how in turn these contributed to the concepts presented in the findings. The reader should be able to follow a clear audit trail of the researchers' decision making throughout the project.

Expert critique adds to a study's auditability and involves the researcher asking others to examine the data and confirm the decision-making process and conclusions made. The 'auditors' may be familiar with the analysis process, have experience in the content area, or use different criteria to examine the data.

Another commonly used validation strategy is the use of *member checking*. This process involves checking the researchers' interpretation against those of the participants. The aim of this process is to reduce possible errors or discrepancies in the reported findings. Member checking may involve activities such as returning transcripts or reports back to participants for confirmation. Despite its conceptual appeal, there may be practical difficulties in asking participants to reflect on information that they have previously provided to the researcher.

Reliability is only used when there are multiple coders on a team who have to reach agreement on codes for a particular piece of qualitative data. The process establishes inter-coder agreement. Several individuals code a transcript using a predetermined coding scheme and then compare their conclusions. Rates are developed for the percentage of codes that are similar, and reliability statistics (Kappas) can be computed for systematic data comparisons.

Use of a *negative case* is an attempt to find disconfirming evidence in the form of information that is contrary to the one established by the inductive analytical process. Such information is used to refine the analysis until it can explain and make sense of the majority of findings.

The *relevance* of the study and its findings can be established through a researcher showing how they contribute to a current body of knowledge. To achieve this, the study needs to be written up in sufficient detail for the findings to be generalised beyond the setting of the study itself; a reader needs enough information to be able to judge whether or not the findings apply or 'fit' in similar settings (*transferability*). Relevance can also be enhanced by the use of probability sampling to ensure that interview participants come from a range of settings that are representative of the wider population (quota or stratified samples).

The overall aim of validation strategies in positivist/postpositivist mixed methods research is to ensure the accuracy of the data collection and analysis processes within both the quantitative and qualitative component. The triangulation of the findings enables the generalisability of the findings. The focus in this paradigm remains on the rigour of what the researcher is doing and its trustworthiness and not on the personal, theoretical and methodological trustworthiness (the thinking and related actions) of the researcher themselves.

Interpretivist/constructivist validation strategies

Although there is a variety of interpretive methodologies, they share a common aim – to come to some understanding or 'truth' of a situation through the self-understandings of participants (Grant and Giddings 2002). In postpositivist qualitative research, participants' experiences are described as accurately as possible through shared agreement. In contrast, an interpretive researcher uses a theoretical framework to interpret the significance of the participants' self-understandings. The outcome of this is that the interpretation may not necessarily accord with those understandings. The researcher acts as a listener and interpreter of the data 'given' by the participant; the researcher's interpretation is brought to the fore in the analysis process. In order to credibly interpret a participant's story, therefore, the researcher needs to understand and make explicit their position in relation to the phenomenon under scrutiny. This requires a degree of self-reflexivity. Although some of the strategies for ensuring the trustworthiness in positivist/ postpositivist qualitative research can be applied to interpretive research, the focus is more on their application in relation to the researcher, rather than on the processes used.

Trustworthiness of the researcher: self-reflexivity

Self-reflexivity involves processes of ensuring the integrity and credibility of the interpretive researcher. The researcher needs to be sensitive to the ways in which they themselves, in terms of their experience and prior assumptions, and the theoretical and methodological processes they have chosen, shape the data collection and analysis. The researcher's pre-understandings, including their beliefs, values and personal biases about the issue being researched, need to be made plain at the outset of a study. One way to develop such self-awareness involves the researcher being interviewed in depth by another qualitative researcher skilled in the chosen methodology. After transcribing the interview, the researcher analyses the data to uncover their pre-understandings. These are then written up in the study and may become integral to the researcher's interpretation of the data. Self-awareness can also be enhanced by good record keeping of the content and processes of communications, including personal reactions to various events.

Also under scrutiny are the researcher's experience and understanding of the interpretive methodology that they are using. In the research report a researcher needs to show how the theoretical components of their methodology were played out in the conduct of the research. For example, in a grounded theory study a researcher can use examples of memos written during the process of the study to show how decisions were made concerning the sampling process in relation to early findings and emergent theory (*theoretical sampling*). This reporting of how the theoretical components of a methodology were applied also facilitates the auditability of a study, which in turn contributes to the overall *credibility* of a study's findings.

In interpretive research, an important validation of a study or its *confirmability* is whether or not the findings are meaningful and applicable in terms of a reader's own experiences (*fittingness*) or extend their understanding or personal constructions of a phenomenon being studied (*authenticity*). For example, if a phenomenological approach is used for the qualitative component of a mixed methods study, a measure of the validity of the study's findings is the 'phenomenological nod' – a person nods in recognition of an experience.

When a mixed methods study involves an interpretive/constructivist methodology, the quantitative component is more likely to be complementary, adding value to the interpretation of the qualitative component. Or in the reporting each takes a complementary position to the other, in other words the mixed methods study produces two different papers, probably published in different but methodologically appropriate journals.

Although the findings of mixed methods studies from within the interpretive/constructivist paradigm are not generalisable in the positivist sense, they are transferable to samples that share certain characteristics or studies that are similar in their settings. *Transferability* of findings is also a feature of validation strategies used in mixed methods research within the critical/radical and poststructural/postmodern paradigms.

Critical/radical validation strategies: situated trustworthiness

Critical/radical (including feminist) research aims to both criticise and change injustices which pervade the social world (Grant and Giddings 2002). Ideally, this kind of research empowers people who suffer from injustice or inequities to act collectively with the researcher to change their circumstances. Critical/radical research, then, is explicitly political. While qualitative methods are more commonly used, mixed methods enquiry has a place. The inclusion of quantitative methods allows us to make certain kinds of arguments about the dominance or not of particular social practices. For instance, feminist educational researchers have used counts of the number of images of boys or men in school textbooks to make arguments about gender bias in curricula (Alton-Lee and Densem 1992). Additionally, quantitative methods are useful for studies that want to gather information from very large groups of people. Such studies have been the foundation of many health sociology projects that have been attentive to gender and race (Weitz 2001).

Given the political agenda of critical/radical research, it is clear that the processes for validating the trustworthiness of such research will need to be significantly different from those required by the previous paradigms. Somewhat confusingly, however, many of the key terms used to describe validation processes in critical/radical and interpretivist/constructivist research are the same. Yet, on closer inspection, we can see their meanings have shifted in important ways.

Situated trustworthiness

The meaning of trustworthiness shifts considerably in this political paradigm. Here, trustworthiness requires that the researcher must have a sharp awareness of their own standpoint – particularly in relation to politics, history and culture. Self-reflexivity is now essential, so that a common strategy in writing about this kind of research has been to open with an account of the researcher's own position and commitments, often through autobiography, including sometimes their theoretical commitments. The process of positioning oneself as a researcher means that the general idea of trustworthiness resolves into a more specific notion of interested or 'situated' trustworthiness.

Validity redefined

The idea of validity likewise undergoes a series of transformations. Lather (1986), an early and influential writer on this topic, talks about 'reconceptualising validity' (p. 67) and suggests that the following guidelines will be useful. First, triangulation needs to be extended beyond the idea of multiple measures to 'include multiple data sources, methods, and theoretical schemes' (Lather 1986: 67). Further, the point of credible triangulation is that the research design seeks 'counter patterns' (Lather 1986: 67) as well as the convergence that is sought in the postpositivist and interpretivist paradigms.

Secondly, Lather (1986) argues that validity in 'openly ideological research' (p. 63) requires three forms: construct validity, face validity and catalytic validity. Construct and face validity have already been discussed in relation to the previous paradigms but here they have a distinctive interpretation and application that is consistent with the critical/radical stance of the research. *Construct validity* means that the researcher must not only account for their research constructs but also acknowledge where those constructs come from. This includes exposing the researcher's theoretical assumptions and standpoint as an active meaning-making force within the research. The researcher must also account for the ways in which key constructs shift during the research in response to the 'logic of the data' (Lather 1986).

Face validity refers to the extent of agreement between the researched and the researcher's interpretations and conclusions. As in the previous paradigms, it is ensured through processes of member checking. However, in many radical/critical research designs, especially those that describe themselves as participatory, participants are part of the research process from beginning to end, including in recurrent cycles of data interpretation. Participants' views of the conclusions that the researcher draws from the study are intimately important for the project's outcomes. In this context, member checking is not so much about accuracy as it is about the full engagement of the research participants with the enquiry process and its consequences.

Finally, *catalytic validity* refers to the extent to which the research contributes to social change. This is in direct contrast to the political neutrality aspired to in positivism/postpositivism and interpretivism/constructivism. Because critical/radical research is committed to social change, the actual changes that result are important measures of the quality of the research. Lather (1986) argues that all three forms of validity are necessary in order to 'protect our research and theory construction from our enthusiasms' (p. 67) and to ensure data credibility.

Various tensions may arise in critical/radical research over differing interpretations of the data. Analyses formed by the researcher may differ from the views of the researched. This is theoretically acceptable because critical social theory suggests that people's experience is often mystified to them through ideology: we may not understand the deeper, structural significance of our personal experience. For example, individual women participants may not understand how the 'fact' of their gender contributes to their unequal positioning within society. Therefore, if a researcher draws conclusions based on this insight, they may well disagree. If this happens, it creates problems for the application of face validity. A researcher may respond by incorporating a participant's views within their theoretical model and/or rethink their assumptions and/or key constructs. Such cycles are characteristic of radical/critical research processes.

Poststructuralist/postmodern validation strategies

The assumption that no one can stand outside the social meanings or worldviews (discourses) of their time underpins research in the post-structuralist/postmodern paradigm (Grant and Giddings 2002). The poststructuralist/postmodern researcher's aim is to explore the way that power works systematically through discourses in order to produce the categories and subject positions of human experience. Such an analysis puts into question the apparent naturalness of the ways in which we make sense of our experience and conduct our lives, such as through the social positions of 'nurse' or 'doctor' or even 'woman' or 'man'. As a consequence, the researcher hopes to disrupt existing patterns in the circulation of meaning and power and to transform and multiply the available discourses and possible subject positions (Jones 1993). Poststructuralist/postmodern enquiry shares the critical/radical impulse to bring about change in the social world, but credible research projects will always be necessarily local and small scale, partial and subjective, even contradictory, because meanings are 'multiple, unstable and open to interpretation' (McCouat and Peile 1995: 10).

In poststructuralist/postmodern enquiry, qualitative methods pre-dominate but are used in especially intensive ways: small amounts of text can form the basis for extended analysis. In this paradigm, 'text' refers to images, architecture, music, body art and clothing as well as the spoken or written word; multiple modes of text might be mixed in one study. Although quantitative methods are rarely used in this context, they could be. For example, counting instances of the use of a word, phrase or image in textual data might provide evidence for making a case for the dominance of a particular discourse.

Validity as 'framings'

The issues of validating research carried out within this paradigm are particularly complex (Lather 2006). While there are continuities with the critical/radical paradigm, there are important differences. For example, the whole question of how knowledge is legitimised is core to this paradigm: knowledge claims are always open to question. Lather (1993) argues that any validity processes applied must be both context-sensitive and open-ended. But, the puzzled researcher might ask, what do such processes look like? Lather (1993) goes on to describe four 'framings' from within which to think about validity: ironic validity, neo-pragmatic validity, rhizomatic validity and situated validity. On examination, they turn out to be elusive and intensely abstract, characterised by adjectives such as these: 'multiple, partial, endlessly deferred' (Lather 1993: 675). Even as she offers her framings, Lather (1993) says they are 'more problem than solution' (p. 683). In closing we argue that the call for specificity in validity practices that emerges in the critical/radical paradigm becomes more acute within the post-structural/postmodern one: the responsibility for the researcher is to be very attentive to validation throughout and to be as transparent about their standpoint and decisions as possible in their accounts of the research. Despite the complexity of validation within this paradigm, a mixed methods technique can usefully be incorporated in poststructural/postmodern research designs because it opens up for scrutiny gaps, contradictions and omissions.

Conclusion

We have argued that health and social sciences research emerges from several distinctive research paradigms and that each requires different approaches to meet expectations of validation. Understanding what counts as robust validation strategies within a given paradigm requires us to understand the underpinning assumptions and beliefs that shape that research worldview. Along the way we have pointed out the continuities that exist between validation processes across paradigms as well as the differences between them. Validation strategies within mixed methods research that is situated within a given paradigm rather than across paradigms, will pose fewer challenges for the researcher. When there are gaps or contradictions within mixed methods research findings, however, they can open up the possibility of developing further questions or hypotheses that may better assist in addressing complex health issues and also herald new methodologies and creative combinations of methods.

References

Alton-Lee A. and Densem P. (1992) Towards a gender-inclusive school curriculum: Changing educational practice. In Middleton S. (ed.) *Women and Education in Aotearoa*, pp. 197–220. Wellington: Bridget Williams.

Creswell J.W. and Plano Clark V.L. (2007) *Designing and Conducting Mixed Methods Research*. Thousand Oaks, CA: Sage.

Giddings L.S. (2006) Mixed methods research: positivism dressed in drag? *Journal of Research in Nursing*, **11**(3), 195–203.

Giddings L.S. and Grant B.M. (2007) A trojan horse for positivism? A critique of mixed methods. *Advances in Nursing Science*, **30**, 52–60.

Giddings L.S. and Williams L.A. (2006) A challenge to the postpositivist domination of mixed methods research: A review of nursing journals 1998–2005. Paper presented at: *The Mixed Methods Conference 2006*, 8–11 July 2006, Cambridge, UK.

Grant B.M. and Giddings L.S. (2002) Making sense of methodologies: a paradigm framework for the novice researcher. *Contemporary Nurse*, **13**(1), 10–28.

Jones A. (1993) Becoming a 'girl': post-structuralist suggestions for educational research. *Gender and Education*, **5**(2), 157–166.

Lather P. (1986) Issues of validity in openly ideological research: between a rock and a soft place. *Interchange*, **17**(4), 63–84.

Lather P. (1993) Fertile obsession: validity after poststructuralism. *Sociological Quarterly*, **34**(4), 673–693.

Lather P. (2006) Paradigm proliferation as a good thing to think with: teaching research in education as a wild profusion. *International Journal of Qualitative Studies in Education*, **19**(1), 35–57.

Lincoln Y.S. and Guba E.G. (1985) *Naturalistic Inquiry*. Beverly Hills, CA: Sage.

McCouat M. and Peile C. (1995) The micro politics of qualitative research traditions. In *Qualitative Research: Beyond the Boundaries*, pp. 2–16. Fremantle, WA: Curtin University of Technology and Sir Charles Gairdner Hospital.

Patton M.Q. (2002) *Qualitative Research and Evaluation Methods*. Thousand Oaks, California: Sage.

Polit D.F. and Beck C.T. (2006) *Essentials of Nursing Research: Methods, Appraisal and Utilization*. Philadelphia: Lippincott, Williams and Wilkins.

Rumsey N., Clarke A., White P., Wyn-Williams M. and Garlick W. (2004) Altered body image: appearance-related concerns of people with visible disfigurement. *Journal of Advanced Nursing*, **48**(5), 443–453.

Tashakkori A. and Teddlie C. (eds.) (2003) *Handbook of Mixed Methods in Social and Behavioral Research*. Thousand Oaks, California: Sage.

Weitz R. (2001) *The Sociology of Health, Illness, and Health Care: A Critical Approach*, 2nd edition. Arizona: Arizona State University.

Reporting Mixed Methods Projects

Alicia O'Cathain

Learning objectives

After reading this chapter you will have the knowledge to:

a) Understand the challenges of reporting mixed methods research.
b) Consider the issues specific to reporting different designs.
c) Critique reports of mixed methods research.
d) Outline models for reporting mixed methods research.
e) Identify considerations specific to reporting mixed methods dissertations and journal papers.

Introduction

Reporting mixed methods research has been recognised as being a significant challenge (Sandelowski 2003; Johnstone 2004; Bryman 2007). Yet it has not received the same attention in the literature on mixed methods research as other issues such as paradigms, typologies and purposes of combining methods (Creswell and Tashakkori 2007). Given that reports, dissertations, theses and peer-reviewed journal articles are the public face of research and the vehicle for disseminating study findings, it is important that this stage of the research process be explored. This chapter focuses on some of the challenges of reporting mixed methods research and offers practical guidance to researchers and students engaged in this endeavour.

The chapter is shaped by my research background, experience and the philosophical position I adopt around mixed methods research. I am a pragmatic researcher in health services research, a field which historically has employed predominantly quantitative enquiry but one in which mixed methods research is increasingly common (O'Cathain et al. 2007a). I have participated in a number of mixed methods studies including: a combination of a randomised controlled trial and ethnographic study to evaluate a new health technology; a multifaceted evaluation of a new health service; a survey and interview study to explore variation in health care; and a focus group study to develop a questionnaire for a survey of patient views of health services. I have adopted two philosophical positions in my mixed methods research – 'implicit pragmatism', where I gave no explicit thought to philosophical issues, and 'subtle realism', which I will return to later in the chapter (Hammersley 1992).

Challenges of reporting mixed methods research

In the past, few researchers have explicitly written about reporting mixed methods research. However, there is a growing body of literature discussing this issue (Sandelowski 2003; Johnstone 2004; Stange et al. 2006; Creswell and Plano Clark 2007; Creswell and Tashakkori 2007). This literature, either implicitly or explicitly, has identified a number of challenges (Table 8.1).

A lack of templates

Peer-reviewed journal articles are probably the most accessible means of disseminating research to both other researchers and research con-

Table 8.1 Challenges of reporting mixed methods research.

A lack of templates
Ordering the presentation
Style, language and voice
Different audiences
The author
Displaying credibility
Journal word limits

sumers in nursing and health care. The prevailing model is of papers reporting either primary qualitative or quantitative research. Journals themselves may be divided largely on methodological grounds, for example the *Lancet* or *Journal of the American Medical Association* might be characterised as quantitative journals. In contrast, journals such as *Qualitative Health Research*, as the name suggests, exclusively publish qualitative research. In such publications the templates made available to prospective authors are generally of purely quantitative or purely qualitative research. Of course papers describing mixed methods research are increasingly being written and published but the infancy of the paradigm has not allowed researchers to assimilate a pattern, or set of patterns, which they can then draw on within their own work. To further complicate matters, mixed methods researchers can publish a number of separate papers from different components of the one study (Brannen 1992; Morse 2003; Stange et al. 2006; O'Cathain et al. 2007b). In addition to the issues of 'salami slicing' that this raises, separating study findings adds to the lack of templates in the peer-reviewed literature. This has occurred with studies I have been involved with, where the quantitative component (O'Cathain et al. 2002) was published separately from the qualitative one (Stapleton et al. 2002). A further example can be seen in the work of Clendon and Krothe where the quantitative component is published in one journal (Clendon 2004) and the qualitative component in another (Clendon and Krothe 2004). See Box 8.1.

Box 8.1 Point to ponder

Mixed methods research should be driven by the underlying principle that the collection of qualitative and quantitative data will provide the best means to answer the research question. Reporting the results separately without some kind of mixing of the data, in most studies, will reduce the power of the findings.

A related issue is that the current templates for reporting either qualitative or quantitative research become familiar to publishers, authors and readers. The familiar is often seen as being the acceptable model, whilst innovation is frequently viewed with suspicion (Sandelowski 2003). However, innovation is likely to be required when reporting mixed methods studies. One way of dealing with any suspicion around innovation is to acknowledge the convention, justify the need to break with convention and then explain the new approach before going on to use it. As more researchers do this, innovative approaches to reporting mixed methods studies will increasingly become part of the conventional approach to reporting research.

There is, however, a limit to the actions which researchers can take as individual agents. Some structural change is needed. If academic journals are the main source of templates for researchers, then they will need to change to reflect the increasing use of mixed methods research. Researchers may not write mixed methods articles if they are concerned that journals will not accept them (Brewer and Hunter 1989; Wong 2002; Currall and Towler 2003), or if the word count is so low that it prohibits adequate description of both qualitative and quantitative methods and findings (Bryman 2007). Additionally, papers reporting mixed methods research may end up published in journals that will accept the research method, rather than being the most appropriate site for dissemination to the target audience within the health sector. Researchers' concerns may arise from direct experience of attempting to publish mixed methods papers or from perceptions developed through seeing mainly quantitative or qualitative articles published.

The publishing situation appears to be changing. A call for a mixed methods journal (Brewer and Hunter 1989) has been addressed with the recent launch of both the *Journal of Mixed Methods Research* and the *International Journal of Multiple Research Approaches*. The word count of the former journal is up to 10 000 words, which offers scope for full description of all components of a study. This is a major step forward but it is still the case that research needs to be disseminated to professions in health care so that they can consider implementing the findings. Whilst publishing in methodology-specific journals may enable the researcher to publish their work in the public domain, such journals are often not the most effective site for dissemination of material to clinician groups upon which it may impact. Editors of all journals will need to consider drawing up explicit criteria relevant to mixed methods papers if they wish to be inclusive of mixed methods research. Key considerations will be specifying a suitable word count for these papers, and developing reviewers with expertise in mixed methods research. The editors of the journal *Annals of Family Medicine* have started this process with an editorial outlining different approaches to publishing mixed methods research, in which they recognise the need for flexibility from journals in terms of expanding word length requirements (Stange et al. 2006). However, they also recognise that authors need to write succinctly because research findings need to be accessible to health professionals.

Ordering the presentation

When reporting results from mixed methods research, deciding on the order of presentation of the qualitative and quantitative components, and the order of presentation of the data collection, analysis and findings of each component, can cause difficulties (Johnstone 2004). Two formats are possible: a sequential format can display the methods and findings of one component followed by the methods and findings of the other component, or an integrated format can weave both components together (Creswell and Plano Clark 2007). The former model is the easier of the two to write and may even be used in an implicit attempt to avoid fully integrating the qualitative and quantitative findings (Bryman 2007). In fact sequential approaches may be common because they reflect the lack of integration which researchers engage in because they tend to treat different components in a study as if they were separate studies (O'Cathain et al. 2007b). Whilst sequential approaches may be suitable for thesis writing, they would probably not be well accepted in the peer-reviewed literature where there is significant pressure to conform to traditional models of ordering the presentation. It has been suggested that sequential formats should be replaced by integrated writing showing the journey between the two datasets (Bazeley 2003) and discussing the timing of analysis and interpretation between the qualitative and quantitative components (Sandelowski 2003). This 'integrated writing' may require considerable thought and has led Johnstone (2004) to draw a conceptual model of the research process of her mixed methods doctoral thesis, showing the complex iterative inter-relationship between the qualitative and quantitative components of her study and how, for example, the qualitative analysis affected the quantitative analysis.

Style, language and voice

Different formatting styles, language and voice are associated with quantitative and qualitative research (Sandelowski 2003; Johnstone 2004; Creswell and Plano Clark 2007). Scientific reports require the separation of findings and interpretation, and the third-person passive voice (Sandelowski 2003). Qualitative research can involve iterative relationships between sampling and analysis, and analysis and interpretation, and an informal personal voice. Researchers can face the dilemma of which to use in their reports, dissertations or articles. In a study where one method is dominant, the style or voice of that dominant component may be used to write up the whole report (Sandelowski 2003). However, researchers may wish to celebrate the differences of both components and use the style, language and voice associated with each component.

   Paradigms are highly relevant here (see Chapter 2). The objective researcher uses the third person whereas the researcher who acknowledges their influence on the research process may use the first person. Therefore researchers need to incorporate rather than ignore the philosophical stance that they are adopting in their research. Possible approaches include pragmatism (Rorty 1982), using whichever voice or style suits different parts of a report, or subtle realism (Hammersley 1992), which requires acknowledgement of the researcher and some use of the first person throughout any report. However, some methods may be more open to a flexible approach to language and style than others. In the field of health care research, the randomised controlled trial has such a tightly controlled template for reporting (Altman 1996) that researchers could risk a poor quality assessment of their work if they do not adhere to it.

Different audiences

Readers may not know what a mixed methods report or article looks like (Creswell and Plano Clark 2007) and may themselves be divided into 'qualitative and quantitative readers' who bring different experiences, language and expectations to reports of studies, making it a challenge to meet the needs of readers when presenting a mixed methods study (Sandelowski 2003). This separation of different audiences by methodological preference can encourage researchers to report findings of mixed methods studies in a way which excludes one component of a study or uses it minimally (Bryman 2007). However, an alternative approach is for researchers to write reports which are accessible and appealing to mixed audiences, ensuring that they are respectful of diverse communities by not depicting one method as inferior or apologising for a 'lack' in one method (Sandelowski 2003).

It is important to consider the audience for whom a report is being written and their knowledge, ease and familiarity with different methodological approaches. This should shape the reporting by perhaps offering more explanation around the method that is least known to the audience, or by taking a simple descriptive (and therefore accessible) approach to the methods of each component. This may result in tension between the values of the researcher and those of the audience, but a key role of the researcher in reporting is to convince an audience to read, digest and value their work.

Health care professionals, policy makers and consumers are important audiences for research. Another important audience is other researchers. Researchers from a number of disciplines are likely to be involved in any mixed methods study and each may wish to write for a discipline-specific audience or publish in journals which are valued within their research community. Career prospects may be linked to publication in specific journals, particularly those with high impact factors, and this may lead to tension within a research team about the optimal place to publish. The pressure in the academic community to publish regularly may lead to the development of multiple papers describing various aspects of a single study. In particular, a mixed methods study can often be carved into multiple papers. Care must be taken to ensure that the research team remains true to their work and plans publications that optimise the quality rather than quantity of dissemination.

The author

In a research higher degree thesis or dissertation there is only one author. This researcher shapes the report and decides on the order, balance and style within it in consultation with the research supervisors. However, in the final report of a mixed methods study there may be multiple authors, each contributing to different components of the study. Although all members of the team contribute to the report, the lead author must ultimately decide how the study is reported. The methodological preference and knowledge of the lead author may influence the space allocated to different components in the report as a whole, and in key parts of the report such as the abstract and discussion. Decisions may not be agreeable to all members of a team and negotiation and compromise may be required. Ideally, potential publications will be mapped out at the commencement of a mixed methods study by the research team. Such planning should include discussions about the role that various team members will take in each publication and the authorship of resulting papers.

Displaying credibility

A key aspect of communicating the credibility of any study is the data and analysis display – numbers and graphs in quantitative research, and quotes and theory figures in qualitative research – used to display evidence to convince the reader (Sandelowski 2003). Researchers will need to consider the balance of evidence displays when reporting their mixed methods research. This will depend on the balance of methods within a study, for example a quantitatively dominant study is likely to display more tables and graphs than quotes. See Chapter 6 for discussion about the presentation of data.

Journal word limits

The low word limits in some journals were discussed earlier as a challenge to reporting results of mixed methods research (Bryman 2007; Creswell and Plano Clark 2007). It is worth highlighting this issue separately because very strict limits such as 2000 or 3000 words can inhibit description of both qualitative and quantitative methods and findings.

Critiquing mixed methods reports

Whilst peer review of publications provides a filter for study quality, it is still necessary for the reader to critically appraise the quality of each research report. This has led to the construction of quality criteria for reporting some types of studies, for example the CONSORT statement for reporting of randomised controlled trials (Altman 1996) and the QUOROM for reporting systematic reviews (Moher et al. 1999). Judgements made by the reader about the quality of a study are wholly dependent on the quality of the reporting. Poor reporting of methodological details affects the assessment of quality of all types of research (Mays et al. 2005), including mixed methods studies (Bryman 2006a). Given the importance of reporting, researchers may benefit from the development of a CONSORT or QUOROM style statement on the reporting of mixed methods studies. The development of any such statement is dependent on the criteria for undertaking a good mixed methods study. Few attempts have been made to develop these criteria (Caracelli and Riggin 1994), but this is rapidly changing as researchers begin to discuss the important issue of quality in mixed methods research (Teddlie and Tashakkori 2003; Sale and Brazil 2004; Bryman 2006a). A discussion on evaluating the quality of mixed methods research was presented in Chapter 7.

Guidance is available on writing good mixed methods manuscripts (Creswell and Tashakkori 2007) and writing and evaluating mixed methods research (Creswell and Plano Clark 2007). It is easy to assume that good quality reporting of a mixed methods study will only involve descriptions of the methods, findings and interpretation of each of the individual components, and that addressing the quality criteria specific to the individual methods will be sufficient. However, there are additional issues which should be reported for mixed methods research (Creswell and Tashakkori 2007) and these include details of the mixed methods design, the integration between components and the theoretical perspective or philosophical stance adopted throughout the study (Creswell 2003).

Reporting the individual methods

Of course it is essential to describe the methods, analysis and findings of individual components within a study (Creswell and Tashakkori 2007). It will also be necessary to apply quality standards for quantitative research to the quantitative component and standards for qualitative research to the qualitative component (Creswell and Plano Clark 2007). This may be difficult, and even impossible, to achieve in any detail for mixed methods papers where journal word counts are strict. However, the degree of detail required for each component may depend on the design used. If the qualitative and quantitative components have equal status then a fairly detailed description will be required for both. However, a briefer description may be appropriate if a method has been used only in a supporting role within a study.

Reporting the design

Attention to the design of a mixed methods study allows readers to make judgements about the quality of the study in terms of the appropriateness of the design for addressing the research question. Research designs for mixed methods research are discussed in detail in Chapter 3. Any report will need description of, and justification for, the mixed methods design (Creswell 2003; Creswell and Plano Clark 2007). The inclusion of a diagram of the design can be an economical means of conveying information about the design to the reader. Creswell (2003) identifies the key characteristics of any design, including the purpose of combining methods, the priority of each method and the order in which methods are used. When the methods and analysis of individual components are reported they can be linked back to this overall design. Table 8.2 provides an extract from my own doctoral thesis which illustrates how I described and justified the design I used. A less detailed version of this might be required to be included in a report, and a few key sentences only might be required within a journal article.

Reporting the integration

Integration is a key component of any mixed methods study (O'Cathain et al. 2007b). It is vital that the qualitative and quantitative data and findings are brought together to offer a fuller understanding of the issue under study (Creswell and Tashakkori 2007). Despite this there is limited discussion in the literature as to how such integration is

Table 8.2 An example of reporting the mixed methods design in a PhD thesis (O'Cathain 2006).

Justification of design	'The overall research question about how to exploit the potential of mixed methods studies in health services research required multiple methods because the broad question contained two narrower questions. It was clear from the literature review that the health services research community can exploit the potential of mixed methods research by drawing on the variety of characteristics of mixed methods studies and undertaking studies to a high quality. However, it was also clear that researchers may encounter facilitators and barriers to undertaking these studies in practice, which may help or hinder them to exploit this approach. The methods were chosen to best address these different aspects of the overall research question. Documentary analysis was selected as a useful approach to studying the characteristics and quality of mixed methods studies in health services research . . . A quantitative content analysis approach to documentary analysis was chosen to study characteristics and quality in order to identify both gaps in the way in which mixed methods research is used in health services research, and the frequency with which they occur . . . The second aspect of the research question was about what helps and hinders researchers to exploit the potential of mixed methods studies . . . Researchers who have undertaken mixed methods studies in health services research will hold perceptions of how researchers can exploit the potential of mixed methods studies . . . some of the barriers and facilitators may not be obvious to researchers themselves, and they may be context dependent (Bryman 1988). A quantitative approach may be premature before those perceptions and experiences are understood in depth. Qualitative methodology offers a flexible approach which could uncover areas not anticipated at the beginning of the research, and which could access the range and depth of people's opinions more than a survey approach (Pill 1995).'
Description of design	'The design of the empirical study was mixed methods with two distinct components – a quantitative documentary analysis and a qualitative interview study. The purpose of using this mixed methods approach was complementarity, that is, that each component would address a different aspect of the question "how to exploit the potential of mixed methods studies in health services research". Each component had equal status within the study and each had "stand alone" status rather than acting merely in a supplementary role to a dominant component . . . A secondary purpose of the mixing of methods was development, with the studies identified in the documentary analysis acting as a sampling frame for the interview study. The sequence therefore was that the documentary analysis was started first and all 75 studies for which documents were available acted as a sampling frame for the interview study. The data extraction for the documentary analysis was completed in the early stages of the interview study and the assessment of the extent to which the mixed methods aspects of a study were exploited was used to sample further interviewees.'

actually achieved. Bazeley, in Chapter 6, has discussed some innovative strategies for integrating qualitative and quantitative data. It is important for the author to be transparent about where and how integration between methods occurred within a study to allow the reader to make judgements about the appropriateness of the integration and how it was undertaken. For example, if findings from the qualitative and quantitative components of a study are compared then the reader may wish to know who was involved in this process, what techniques – if any – were used, and if attention was paid to contradictory as well as convergent findings. Additionally, such knowledge can provide a model to guide future researchers in designing their mixed methods studies.

Reporting the philosophical stance adopted

Readers are likely to make judgements about the quality of a paper based on their own philosophical positions. Therefore it is important that researchers position themselves explicitly when reporting their research and thereby communicate the quality criteria they wish to be judged by. In my doctoral thesis, which I introduced in Table 8.2, I was explicit that I wanted the quality of my quantitative documentary analysis to be judged using criteria identified for that method, and the quality of my qualitative interviews to be judged using criteria identified for that method. However, I adopted the perspective of subtle realism overall for the whole study. This meant that I had to situate myself within the research and describe how my research experience led me to be interested in particular aspects of my topic and interested in particular ways of researching this topic. I had to recognise that the choices and interpretations I made for both components of my study were shaped by my experience and beliefs. Reporting of one's philosophical position may be essential in doctoral theses, and desirable in dissertations, but may be rarely found in peer-reviewed journal articles. Bryman (2006b) found that only 6% of over 200 mixed methods journal articles published in social research mentioned anything about paradigms. Journal word count limitations may account for this, so when writing mixed methods articles authors may need to consider how essential paradigm statements are to the journal editor and readership as well as to themselves.

Ways of reporting different outputs

A variety of outputs is possible from mixed methods studies – reports for funding bodies, dissertations or theses for degrees and peer-reviewed journal articles. Each type of output holds its own challenges and is discussed below.

Writing reports, dissertations and theses

A book has been written about blending qualitative and quantitative methods in dissertations and theses (Thomas 2003). However, it focuses on writing research proposals and the range of opportunities for publication rather than reporting results. When writing reports, dissertations and theses it is important to consider whether to follow a segregated or integrated model, the language and style to adopt throughout the body of the text, and the order of presentation of the qualitative and quantitative components.

Segregated and integrated models

As part of my doctoral thesis, introduced in Table 8.2, I undertook a study of 75 mixed methods projects funded by the UK Department of Health between 1994 and 2004 (O'Cathain et al. 2007b). Within the completed projects, I identified the two approaches to reporting which I introduced earlier in the chapter – the 'segregated' and 'integrated' models of report writing (Table 8.3). There are various formats of both models.

Table 8.3 Segregated and integrated models of report writing.

Segregated models		Integrated model	
A		Chapter 1	Background
Chapter 1	Background	Chapter 2	Methods (including mixed methods design, quantitative method, qualitative method and description of integration)
Chapter 2	Quantitative methods and results		
Chapter 3	Qualitative methods and findings		
Chapter 4	Long discussion	Chapter 3	Findings: Theme 1 (based on any or all components)
B		Chapter 4	Findings: Theme 2 (based on any or all components)
Chapter 1	Background		
Chapter 2	Methods (quantitative and qualitative)	Chapter 5	Findings: Theme 3 (based on any or all components)
Chapter 3	Quantitative results	Chapter 6	Discussion
Chapter 4	Qualitative findings		
Chapter 5	Discussion		

Table 8.4 Different approaches to writing reports for funding bodies in mixed methods studies funded by the Department of Health in England, 1994–2004.

Dissemination	Report (n = 48)
Segregated model	65% (31)
Integrated model	31% (15)
Not enough information	4% (2)

The segregated model kept the qualitative and quantitative components of a study separate, devoting individual chapters to each. Any integration between components occurred in the discussion of the report only, bringing together the findings or implications from each component for consideration in the final chapter of the report. It was usual for only small amounts of integration to have occurred for a few points only, leaving the potential for considerably more integration between different components (O'Cathain et al. 2007b). Of the two, the segregated model was the most common approach identified (Table 8.4).

The less commonly used approach was the 'integrated model', where findings from the different methods were interwoven within results chapters, each of which focused on one aspect of the research question or research theme. Either the qualitative or quantitative component, or both, were drawn on within each results chapter depending on the contribution each dataset made to the research question or theme under consideration in a chapter.

When I reflect back on the mixed methods reports I have been involved in, I realise that I have always followed a segregated model. For the study I introduced in Table 8.2, methods included a quantitative documentary analysis of 75 mixed methods studies and a qualitative interview study of 20 researchers who had worked on some of these studies. In the early stages of writing up this study I followed the segregated model, where any integration between the qualitative and quantitative components was left to the discussion section of the report. I never got around to writing the discussion of this version but I remember finding the size of the task quite daunting and expected the discussion chapter to be extremely long. As my writing-up progressed, I realised that I was following the reporting mode I had seen commonly within mixed methods reports. However, I wanted to treat my study as a mixed methods endeavour rather than as two separate studies within one. Therefore I restructured the report to an integrated model and this enabled me to address some specific mixed methods issues relevant to good reporting of a mixed methods study (see earlier

Table 8.5 Outline of a segregated and integrated model of the same doctoral thesis.

Integrated model
Chapter 1   Introduction *(including philosophical position)*
Chapter 2   Literature review
Chapter 3   Methods *(including mixed methods design, quantitative method, qualitative method and description of integration)*
Chapter 4   Results *(types of studies, based on quantitative data only)*
Chapter 5   Results *(quality of studies, based on both components)*
Chapter 6   Results *(facilitators and barriers, based on qualitative data only, with discussion)*
Chapter 7   Results *(based on integration between the quantitative and qualitative components)*
Chapter 8   Short discussion
Segregated model
Chapter 1   Introduction
Chapter 2   Literature review
Chapter 3   Quantitative method *(description of documentary analysis)*
Chapter 4   Quantitative results *(types of studies)*
Chapter 5   Quantitative results *(quality of studies)*
Chapter 6   Qualitative methods *(description of interviews)*
Chapter 7   Qualitative findings *(facilitators and barriers to mixed methods studies)*
Chapter 8   Long discussion

section), including a chapter focused on integration of data and findings from the qualitative and quantitative components. Table 8.5 provides outlines of the segregated and integrated models of my doctoral thesis.

Reports based on an integrated model can have any number of results chapters, of varied sizes. For example, a report of a new approach to general practice provision reported all the methods in a methods chapter, followed by six results chapters each covering an aspect of the new service such as patient experience or impact on other providers (Hallam and Henthorpe 1999). Results chapters varied in size from four pages to twelve pages long, and drew either solely on the qualitative data, solely on the quantitative data, or on both. The authors also used findings from early results chapters when reporting findings in later results chapters. Johnstone (2004) describes in detail her approach to designing an integrated doctoral thesis. Similarly to the Hallam and Henthorpe (1999) report, she had results chapters of very different sizes, and integrated qualitative and quantitative findings in results chapters.

Language, style and order

The language and style used in a report can depend on the research and the researcher. Johnstone (2004) used the first person overall in her thesis because this was consistent with the dominant naturalistic paradigm of her study, but used the third person in some chapters such as the literature review, methods and quantitative findings. In my doctoral thesis I decided that my philosophical position was one of subtle realism for the whole study. I acknowledged that I shaped the quantitative documentary analysis as much as the qualitative interviews study. I discussed this in detail in the introduction of the thesis, using the first person. I then adopted the third person for the rest of the thesis, returning to the first person for parts of the discussion. I made this choice because of my research community, where the third person is predominantly used. Whenever I adopted the first person I explained why I was doing so to ensure that the reader knew that I had deliberately decided not to follow my research community's implicit template.

It does not seem sensible to present a template for the order of presentation of qualitative and quantitative methods and findings because this will largely be dictated by the design, findings, level of integration and conclusions. Bazeley (2003) recommends that the presentation follows the logical chain of evidence leading to the conclusions of the study. This may not be completely possible because of the complexities of the interactions between qualitative and quantitative components.

Diagrams can be very useful for communicating the complexity of the study. I felt that it was essential to include a diagram of interactions between components in my doctoral thesis (Figure 8.1).

Even when decisions have been made about the general order in which to present methods and findings, some sections of a report may need to be presented in an order that is unusual in mono-method studies. For example, in an early version of my doctoral thesis I reported the response rate to my quantitative component in the results section. However, I needed this information to be known earlier in the thesis because these responses became the sampling frame for my qualitative interviews. Therefore I chose to report response rates in my methods section. I explicitly identified to the reader that I had deliberately chosen not to follow the usual order to facilitate communication of the study as a whole.

Writing peer-reviewed publications

Types of articles

Before considering mixed methods articles in peer-reviewed journals, it is worth considering the different types of articles which might

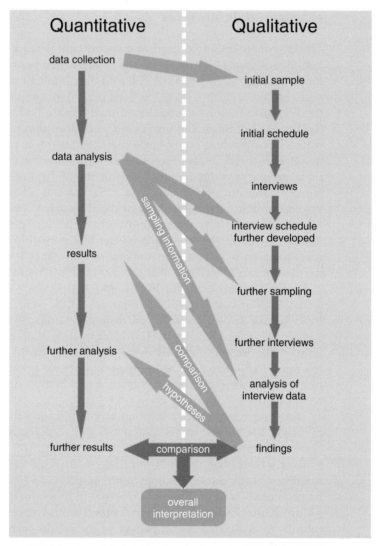

Figure 8.1 Visual model of a mixed methods study (O'Cathain 2006).

emerge from a mixed methods study. Stange et al. (2006) describe five different ways of publishing from a mixed methods study in the context of health research in primary care, and offer examples of them within their journal. Many of them are similar to the types of publications found to emerge from mixed methods studies in health services research (O'Cathain et al. 2007b). One approach to publishing is to report different components of a study in different journals at different times. Doing this without one paper making reference to the other paper does occur, and would seem to defeat the objective of mixed methods research which has a purpose of offering a wider picture of the phenomenon under study (O'Cathain et al. 2007b). However, making ample reference to one published article from a study within another article can be very effective. For example, Donovan and colleagues published an article based on the qualitative component of their study (Mills et al. 2003) and then referenced and discussed the findings of this qualitative component in the discussion section of an article based on the quantitative component of their study (Donovan et al. 2003). The qualitative component helped to explain the findings from the quantitative component rather than leave unanswered questions or rely on mere speculation on the part of the researchers. Whilst such presentation is alluring to the researcher, it may draw criticism from journal editorial boards who may perceive this as salami slicing. A second approach to publishing is to report both components side by side in separate papers in the same issue of the same journal. An example of this is a process evaluation based on qualitative methods (Stapleton et al. 2002) published alongside an outcome evaluation of evidence-based leaflets in maternity care (O'Cathain et al. 2002). This at least provides the reader with the wider picture in the paper copy of the journal, although this advantage will be lost when journal articles are searched electronically. Achieving such publication requires close cooperation by the editorial board and appreciation of the value of this strategy to the journal's readership. A third approach is to write an overview paper which draws together the lessons from a range of articles which have emerged from a mixed methods study. An example of this is an article which draws on the final report and four published articles from an evaluation of a new health service (Salisbury 2003). Finally, an approach can be a mixed methods article which reports the methods and findings from both the qualitative and quantitative components of a study.

Researchers can attempt to report the whole, or almost all of a study in a single mixed methods article. As discussed earlier, this may be challenging in the context of current author guidelines. Alternatively researchers can focus on one aspect of a study only in a mixed methods article, where this is one of a number of articles emerging from a study, and where other papers focus on one component of a study only. The advantage of this latter approach is that all the detailed methods of both components do not have to be covered within one paper. An example of this is a mixed methods study of nurse telephone triage which had a quantitative and a qualitative component occurring concurrently with equal status (O'Cathain et al. 2004b). The quantitative component was undertaken to identify the characteristics of nurses which affected the triage decision made using computerised decision support software. A survey of hundreds of nurses was undertaken to identify their characteristics; this was combined with routine data on the triage decision made by these nurses. The qualitative component, of 24 interviews with nurses, was set up to explore the decision-making processes of nurses. We decided to publish a paper based solely on the qualitative component first. This explored nurses' accounts of their use of the software and how nurses could influence the triage decision when using the software (O'Cathain et al. 2004b). We felt it was important to document first that nurses could influence the triage decision and how they could do this both explicitly and implicitly. We then wrote a second paper – a mixed methods article – within the 5000-word limit set by the journal for qualitative articles (O'Cathain et al. 2004a). The qualitative methods were summarised in this paper with reference made to the detailed methods published in the first paper. This allowed more space for reporting the findings from both components.

Creswell and Plano Clark (2007) give a very helpful outline of the structure of a mixed methods article. Mixed methods articles can be written in a segregated or integrated model in the same way as reports. The mixed methods article from the nurse triage study described above followed a segregated model. In Table 8.6 I describe some key features of this article and some of the decisions faced when writing it.

Reporting different study designs

How a researcher chooses to report a study may depend on the specific design used as well as the story that they are trying to communicate (Creswell and Plano Clark 2007). There are so many variants of different designs that it would not be possible to consider how best to report results for all of them. However, key aspects of designs bring specific considerations that can inform the reporting of results.

Designs with the purpose of confirmation, complementarity or development

If the purpose of the study is confirmation then a segregated model of reporting will be essential. Independent data collection and analysis is needed of both components before the findings of each are brought together in the discussion section of a report (Caracelli and Greene 1993). If the purpose is development, for example a qualitative component is undertaken to develop a questionnaire for a quantitative component, then this sequential design may lend itself to a segregated model of reporting. There is much more scope available to the researcher if the purpose of combining is complementarity, where an integrated

Table 8.6 Decisions made when writing a mixed methods article.

The article
O'Cathain A., Nicholl J., Sampson F., Walters S., McDonnell A. and Munro J. (2004a) Do different types of nurses give different triage decisions in NHS Direct? A mixed methods study. *Journal of Health Services Research and Policy*, **9**(4), 226–233.

Language
Third person throughout. This was an implicit decision and reflects the background of the first author which is grounded in quantitative research.

Methods section
We began the methods with an overview section stating the roles of the two components, and the timing of the components. The relationship between them was that early analysis of the qualitative component identified hypotheses to test in the quantitative component and then the completed qualitative analysis illuminated and explained the quantitative findings.
Then the methods of the two components were described separately. They had been undertaken in a broadly concurrent way so we had to make a decision about which to report first. Although the main role of the qualitative component in the paper was to illuminate findings of the quantitative component, the quantitative component had been informed by preliminary analysis of the qualitative component. Therefore we decided to describe the qualitative component first. The description of the methods was not balanced between the two components – one paragraph to three – because we were able to reference a previous paper from the same study which reported the qualitative methods.

Results section
The order of presentation of the findings was hard to work out until we realised that we could follow the iterative approach of the study, that is, summarise a key finding from the previously published qualitative component, then present the quantitative results in four paragraphs with three tables displaying the data and multilevel model, and then present the qualitative results in six themes with supporting quotes. The balance was one and a half pages for the quantitative results and two pages for the qualitative results.
In the draft accepted by the journal editors we had presented some of the findings from the qualitative component in the context of supporting literature because we felt this helped us to communicate our findings and conclusions. However the sub-editor asked us to remove this to the discussion section of the paper.

Discussion
In the discussion we interpreted both sets of findings. First, we summarised the findings from the quantitative component in three paragraphs and embedded them in the wider literature. Note that this did not follow the order in which the methods were presented. This lack of consistency felt uncomfortable but we concluded that it suited the telling of the story within the paper. Then we summarised the findings from the qualitative component in one paragraph and embedded them in the literature. Then we considered integration. Although the purpose of combining the two components was complementarity rather than confirmation, one of the reviewers of the paper felt that the qualitative and quantitative findings seemed to contradict each other and we considered this in the final draft accepted by the editors.

Level of integration
On reflection, further integration could have been achieved by reporting the findings together, for example by drawing on the qualitative and quantitative findings to consider the effect of each characteristic of nurses on triage outcomes. This more integrated approach to reporting may have identified further analyses for us to undertake and pushed us to identify further insights.

model may be more fruitful. In some studies there may be more than one purpose of combining methods. For example, in my doctoral thesis, the two components were combined mainly for the purpose of complementarity, but the quantitative component also had the purpose of development by acting as a sampling frame for the qualitative component. Reporting these more complex studies will require creativity on the part of researchers, informed by the story the researcher is communicating within the report.

Dominant or equal designs

As previously discussed, if one component of a study is dominant then it seems sensible to let this method govern the reporting in terms of taking up more pages in a report or paragraphs in an article, and determining the voice and language used throughout the write-up (Sandelowski 2003). However, prior to making this decision, it is important to consider how supplementary the non-dominant component is. If it is merely in a supporting role, for example some semi-structured interviews are undertaken with the sole aim of identifying items and language for a questionnaire for use in a survey which is the focus of the study, then this will work. However, even though it is not the main focus of the study, a component may have standalone status. For example, the aim of the semi-structured interviews in the example above may also be to address a research question in their own right. In this case, the researcher may decide to use a different language and style when reporting each component. Even if components have equal status within a study, this may not be the case for any papers emerging from the study. For some papers emerging from a study, one component may be dominant because of the aspect of the research question the researcher is addressing within the paper.

Sequential or concurrent designs

When methods are undertaken in sequence one might expect a study to be reported in two distinct phases, following the order of the data collection. If a qualitative component has been undertaken first, then one would expect it to be reported first, followed by the quantitative component. However, just because data collection has been undertaken in one sequence does not mean that analyses are undertaken in that sequence, or that this sequence dictates the way in which the findings contribute to the conclusions. It may be the case that the researcher may work iteratively between the components of a study as it progresses. For example, in my doctoral thesis, I undertook the quantitative component first because it acted as a sampling frame for my qualitative component. Following this order, I described the quantitative methods before the qualitative methods, and reported the majority of the findings from the quantitative component before those from the qualitative component. However, I considered qualitative and quantitative findings together and reported them together for some themes within my thesis. I also returned to the quantitative component of my study in a later chapter because the findings from the qualitative component directed further analysis of the quantitative data.

The order of reporting is not obvious for concurrent designs and the same issues apply here as with sequential designs. Even in concurrent designs some data collection for one component may occur before the other. The order of data collection may be important in determining the order of presentation but, as before, it is recommended that researchers take a creative approach to considering how best to communicate the story of the research findings and conclusions drawn rather than simply follow the simple order of data collection.

Conclusion

This chapter started with a statement that reporting mixed methods studies is a challenge. I think it is a challenge that we should welcome and enjoy as researchers because it requires creativity when attending to order of presentation, voice and format within our writing up. It is important to know who will read and make judgements about our research, and write with them in mind. It is likely that reporting results from mixed methods research will require some novel approaches, and it will be important for researchers to understand when they are doing something novel from the perspective of the target audience and let them know that an explicit decision has been made to break with convention. Researchers need to actively engage in discussions with editorial boards to develop strategies which optimise the dissemination of mixed methods research.

Reporting mixed methods studies is about more than simply reporting the methods and findings from a qualitative and a quantitative component. Attention is required to the aspects of a study which are unique to mixed methods research, that is, justifying the need for mixed methods research and the combination of methods proposed, describing the combination used and describing the integration. Using a segregated model of reporting may be an automatic response but an integrated model may lead to a more sophisticated report and a higher yield in terms of the insights gained.

A mixed methods study does not have to result in a mixed methods article which covers the whole study. A number of papers can emerge from each project, some of which are based on one component only. However, at least some of the papers should address integration between different components of a study. Otherwise one needs to ask why a mixed methods study was undertaken in the first place. Mixed methods research has the potential to achieve more complete answers to some research questions than mono-method designs. Let us take up the challenge of reporting them in ways which communicate the unique insights which may be available to this approach.

References

Altman D.G. (1996) Better reporting of randomised controlled trials: the CONSORT statement. *British Medical Journal*, **313**, 570–571.

Bazeley P. (2003) Computerized data analysis for mixed methods research. In Tashakkori A. and Teddlie C. (eds.) *Handbook of Mixed Methods in Social and Behavioral Research*, pp. 385–422. London: Sage Publications.

Brannen J. (1992) Combining qualitative and quantitative approaches: an overview. In Brannen J. (ed.) *Mixing Methods: Qualitative and Quantitative Research*, pp. 3–38. Aldershot: Ashgate.

Brewer J. and Hunter A. (1989) *Multimethod Research*. London: Sage Publications.

Bryman A. (1988) *Quantity and Quality in Social Research*. London: Routledge.

Bryman A. (2006a) Paradigm peace and the implications for quality. *International Journal of Social Research Methodology*, **9**, 111–126.

Bryman A. (2006b) Integrating quantitative and qualitative research: how is it done? *Qualitative Research*, **6**, 97–113.

Bryman A. (2007) Barriers to integrating quantitative and qualitative research. *Journal of Mixed Methods Research*, **1**(1), 8–22.

Caracelli V.J. and Greene J.C. (1993) Data analysis strategies for mixed-method evaluation designs. *Educational Evaluation and Policy Analysis*, **15**(2), 195–207.

Caracelli V.J. and Riggin L.J.C. (1994) Mixed-method evaluation: developing quality criteria through concept mapping. *Evaluation Practice*, **15**(2), 139–152.

Clendon J. (2004) Demonstrating outcomes in a nurse-led clinic: how primary health care nurses make a difference to children and their families. *Contemporary Nurse*, **18**(1/2), 164–176.

Clendon J. and Krothe J. (2004) The nurse-managed clinic: an evaluative study. *Nursing Praxis in New Zealand*, **20**(2), 15–23.

Creswell J.W. (2003) *Research Design. Qualitative, Quantitative, and Mixed Methods Approaches*, 2nd edition. London: Sage Publications.

Creswell J.W. and Plano Clark V. (2007) *Designing and Conducting Mixed Methods Research*. Thousand Oaks, California: Sage Publications.

Creswell J.W. and Tashakkori A. (2007) Developing publishable mixed methods manuscripts. *Journal of Mixed Methods Research*, **1**(2), 107–111.

Currall S.C. and Towler A.J. (2003) Research methods in management and organizational research: toward integration of qualitative and quantitative techniques. In Tashakkori A. and Teddlie C. (eds.) *Handbook of Mixed Methods in Social and Behavioral Research*, pp. 513–525. London: Sage Publications.

Donovan J.L., Peters T.J., Noble S., Powell P., Gillat D., Oliver S.R. et al. (2003) Who can best recruit to randomised trials? Randomised trial comparing surgeons and nurses recruiting patients to a trial of treatments for localized prostate cancer (the ProtecT study). *Journal of Clinical Epidemiology*, **56**, 605–609.

Hallam L. and Henthorpe K. (1999) Cooperatives and their primary care emergency centres: organisation and impact. *Health Technology Assessment*, **3**(7), http://www.hta.ac.uk/fullmono/mon307.pdf.

Hammersley M. (1992) *What's Wrong with Ethnography?* London: Routledge.

Johnstone P.L. (2004) Mixed methods, mixed methodology health services research in practice. *Qualitative Health Research*, **14**(2), 259–271.

Mays N., Pope C. and Popay J. (2005) Systematically reviewing qualitative and quantitative evidence to inform management and policy-making in the health field. *Journal of Health Services Research and Policy*, **10**(Suppl 1), 6–20.

Mills N., Donovan J.L., Smith M., Jacoby A., Neal D.E. and Hamdy F.C. (2003) Perceptions of equipoise are crucial to trial participation: a qualitative study of men in the ProtecT study. *Controlled Clinical Trials*, **24**, 272–282.

Moher D., Cook D.J., Eastwood S., Olkin I., Rennie D. and Stroup D.F. (1999) Improving the quality of reports of meta-analyses of randomised controlled trials: The QUOROM statement. *Lancet*, **354**, 1896–1900.

Morse J.M. (2003) Principles of mixed methods and multimethod research design. In Tashakkori A. and Teddlie C. (eds.) *Handbook of Mixed Methods in Social and Behavioral Research*, pp. 189–208. London: Sage Publications.

O'Cathain A. (2006) *Exploiting the Potential of Mixed Methods Studies in Health Services Research*. Unpublished Doctoral thesis, School of Health and Related Research, University of Sheffield.

O'Cathain A., Murphy E. and Nicholl J. (2007a) Why, and how, mixed methods research is undertaken in health services research: a mixed methods study. *BMC Health Services Research*, **7**, 85.

O'Cathain A., Murphy E. and Nicholl J. (2007b) Integration and publications as indicators of 'yield' from mixed methods studies. *Journal of Mixed Methods Research*, **1**(2), 147–163.

O'Cathain A., Nicholl J., Sampson F., Walters S., McDonnell A. and Munro J. (2004a) Do different types of nurses give different triage decisions in NHS Direct? A mixed methods study. *Journal of Health Services Research and Policy*, **9**(4), 226–233.

O'Cathain A., Sampson F.C., Munro J.F., Thomas K.J. and Nicholl J.P. (2004b) Nurses' views of using computerized decision support software in NHS Direct. *Journal of Advanced Nursing*, **45**(3), 280–286.

O'Cathain A., Walters S.J., Nicholl J.P., Thomas K.J. and Kirkham M. (2002) Use of evidence based leaflets to promote informed choice in maternity care: randomised controlled trial in everyday practice. *British Medical Journal*, **324**, 643–646.

Pill R. (1995) Fitting the method to the question; the quantitative or qualitative approach? In Jones R. and Kinmonth A.L. (eds.) *Critical Reading for Primary Care*, pp. 42–58. Oxford: Oxford University Press.

Rorty R. (1982) Pragmatism, relativism, and irrationalism. In Rorty R. (ed.) *Consequences of Pragmatism*, pp. 160–175. Minneapolis: University of Minnesota Press.

Sale J.E.M. and Brazil K. (2004) A strategy to identify critical appraisal criteria for primary mixed method studies. *Quality and Quantity*, **38**(4), 351–365.

Salisbury C. (2003) Do NHS walk-in centres in England provide a model of integrated care? *International Journal of Integrated Care*, **3**, http://www.ijic.org/.

Sandelowski M. (2003) Tables or tableaux? The challenges of writing and reading mixed methods studies. In Tashakkori A. and Teddlie C. (eds.) *Handbook of Mixed Methods in Social and Behavioral Research*, pp. 321–350. London: Sage Publications.

Stange K.C., Crabtree B.F. and Miller W.L. (2006) Publishing multimethod research. *Annals of Family Medicine*, **4**(4), 292–294.

Stapleton H., Kirkham M. and Thomas G. (2002) Qualitative study of evidence based leaflets in maternity care. *British Medical Journal*, **324**, 639–643.

Teddlie C. and Tashakkori A. (2003) Major issues and controversies in the use of mixed methods in the social and behavioural sciences. In Tashakkori A. and Teddlie C. (eds.) *Handbook of Mixed Methods in Social and Behavioral Research*, pp. 3–50. London: Sage Publications.

Thomas R.M. (2003) *Blending Qualitative and Quantitative Research Methods in Theses and Dissertations*. Thousand Oaks, California: Corwin Press.

Wong W. (2002) Did how we learn affect what we learn? Methodological bias, multimethod research and the case of economic development. *Social Science Journal*, **39**, 247–264.

Section Three

Exemplars of Mixed Methods Research

Mixed Methods Intervention Trials

John W. Creswell, Michael D. Fetters, Vicki L. Plano Clark, Alejandro Morales

Learning objectives

The aim of this chapter is to explore the use of mixed methods research designs, incorporating qualitative data collection and analysis, in intervention trials. By the end of this chapter, you will have the knowledge to:

a) Understand the value of adding qualitative data to an intervention trial.
b) Describe strategies useful for incorporating qualitative data into three major types of mixed methods intervention trial designs.
c) Visually illustrate the use of qualitative data in intervention trials.

Introduction

In health sciences research, significant methodological diversity of clinical research has occurred during the past two decades (Stange et al. 2006). Indeed, Borkan (2004) considers mixed methods research as a 'foundation for primary care research' (p. 4). In both the health and social sciences, the increased popularity of mixed methods research is partly due to the gradual acceptance of qualitative approaches, and the tacit recognition that the voices of participants, their context and

the complexity of their narratives can add substantially to the understanding of research problems based on trends, frequencies and statistical relationships in quantitative research. Calls for incorporating
qualitative data in health science research (Rogers et al. 2003) have
been published in several prestigious health journals, including the
Lancet (Malterud 2001), *Journal of the American Medical Association*
(Giacomini and Cook 2000), the *British Medical Journal* (Donovan et al.
2002) and *Journal of Palliative Medicine* (Wallen and Berger 2004). US
federal agencies such as the National Institutes of Health (1999), the
National Science Foundation and the National Research Council have
issued guidelines or provided workshops supporting both qualitative
and mixed methods research (Creswell and Plano Clark 2006). Despite
these endorsements, the potential for incorporating qualitative data in
quantitative health science investigations is still being explored (Borkan
2004).

The purpose of this chapter is to explore one approach to mixing
methods in the health sciences, the use of qualitative research in intervention trials. With embedded qualitative data collection, intervention
trials become a mixed methods research design. For clarity, throughout
this chapter these studies will be referred to as 'mixed methods intervention designs'. An intervention trial is an experimental study in
which the researcher uses procedures to determine whether a treatment influences an outcome (Creswell 2008). This exploration of the
use of qualitative data in intervention trials began with an assessment
of the design characteristics of mixed methods studies in primary
health care. During this assessment, the authors found a study in which
qualitative data augmented the results of an intervention trial
(Baskerville et al. 2001). This finding led to a more detailed examination
of this mixed methods design which revealed a framework to assist in
conceptualisation of this type of study (Sandelowski 1996). With this
conceptualisation in mind, the authors then sought out exemplars of
published studies that illustrated such mixed methods intervention
trials in the health science literature. This chapter presents these steps
in the process of conceptualising and finding mixed methods intervention studies.

Mixed methods designs in primary care

Creswell et al. (2004) examined the mixed methods research designs
being reported in primary health care. A MEDLINE search of the literature published between 1990 and 2001 was used to identify relevant
studies. Relevant studies met the inclusion criteria of incorporating
both quantitative and qualitative data collection and analysis, mixing

or combining the data at some stage in the process of research, focusing on primary care settings, and evidence-based studies reported as single articles in health science publications. Next, the included articles were analysed using criteria for critiquing mixed methods studies that had been derived from the social sciences in such diverse fields as applied psychology, physics education and the social sciences (Hanson et al. 2005; Plano Clark 2005). The criteria included noting the authors' rationale for mixing, the forms of quantitative and qualitative data collected and analysed and the major characteristics of the designs (such as priority for one form of data or the other, the timing of the data collection and the stage in which mixing occurred). The authors also noted the type of design that had been employed using design types specified in analyses of mixed methods studies in the social and behavioural sciences (Creswell et al. 2003).

From the larger pool of mixed methods studies that met the inclusion criteria, the authors selected five studies to analyse in depth (McVea et al. 1996; Kutner et al. 1999; Baskerville et al. 2001; McIlvain et al. 2002; Nutting et al. 2002). From this analysis three designs were identified that the primary care researchers had employed in their studies. Although the researchers did not present diagrams of the procedures for these designs in their publications, Figure 9.1 presents visual models of the general procedures used in each of the three designs (Creswell et al. 2004).

The first design, called the instrument design model, was a mixed methods approach in which the researchers first collected qualitative

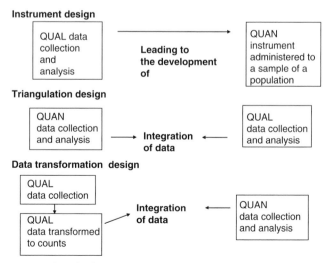

Figure 9.1 Mixed methods intervention designs used in primary care (Creswell et al. 2004).

data, analysed it and then used the findings to develop a quantitative instrument that was, in turn, administered to a sample. This design was illustrated by Kutner et al.'s (1999) primary care study of terminally ill patients and their care. This study involved gathering qualitative, face-to-face interview data in the first phase, analysing the data for codes and themes and then using the findings to design a multiple choice and open-ended question survey instrument, which was subsequently administered to a relevant population sample.

The second design, called the triangulation design model, involved collecting both quantitative and qualitative data simultaneously and then merging the results for a comprehensive understanding of the research problem. The development of case profiles of family practices, incorporating both qualitative and quantitative elements, that differed in terms of their effectiveness of prevention programmes illustrated this design (McVea et al. 1996).

The third design, the data transformation design model, involved collecting qualitative data, converting it to numerical data by counting codes or themes and then comparing the numerical data with quantitative data gathered on instruments. McIlvain et al. (2002) used this design in their study of factors associated with the use of counselling skills and office activities related to tobacco control by family physicians.

The identification of these three models provided a conceptualisation for mixed methods applications in primary care, and these designs added rigour and clarity to complex mixed methods designs used in intervention trials. As a concluding statement, Creswell et al. (2004) noted that future analysis of primary care mixed methods investigations 'might focus on models addressed in the literature but not discussed here' (p. 12).

Mixed methods designs in intervention trials

In addition to the above three designs, there is another model not discussed in the set of five studies. Baskerville et al. (2001) illustrate an evaluation study of 22 intervention practices for implementing prevention guidelines by 54 family physicians. This study not only represented a triangulation design, it also demonstrated a type of design in which qualitative data were concurrently gathered along with quantitative data in an intervention trial. This study led us to consider how qualitative datasets were being introduced by researchers into intervention trials, recognising that intervention trials were often seen as the 'gold standard' of clinical research. At the same time, expansion was occurring in the conceptualisation of the types of mixed methods designs and the utility of a mixed methods approach (Creswell and

Plano Clark 2006). A 'new' type of design was introduced into the social and behavioural science literature – the 'concurrent nested' design (Greene and Caracelli 1997; Creswell et al. 2003). In this design, the researcher emphasised either quantitative or qualitative data and then used the form of data not emphasised in a secondary, supporting role. Morse (1991) had earlier discussed how a primary qualitative design could embed some quantitative data into the research to enrich the description of the sample participants. In contrast, a more common approach in the health sciences literature was to embed a secondary qualitative method (e.g. focus groups) within a larger, primary quantitative data collection (e.g. experimental trial). Some qualitative researchers have felt that such a design relegates and marginalises qualitative research to secondary status (Howe 2004). However, a counterargument is that it serves to encourage the use of qualitative research within the broader forum of quantitative research, and that this added utility of qualitative data far outweighs any secondary status that may be perceived about the qualitative arm of a study (Creswell et al. 2006). The authors were also aware of feedback on several proposals written for private foundations and for US federal agencies in which programme officers encouraged the use of qualitative data to enhance proposed experimental designs.

Finally, the authors began to focus on a definition of mixed methods research that was actually based on evidence-based practice. Mixed methods research, in this definition, became a means for conducting research designs. For example, mixing methods is a means for conducting research within a narrative study (Eliot 2005), a case study (Luck et al. 2006), a correlational study (Harrison 2007) or an experimental investigation (Sandelowski 1996). Thus, mixed methods procedures involving the collection of both quantitative and qualitative data can be incorporated into traditional health sciences epidemiological methods, such as randomised controlled trials, correlational (observational) research and cross-sectional prevalence studies or case control retrospective studies (these methods are reviewed by Marvel et al. (1991)). From among these health science methods, the focus here will be on experimental designs inasmuch as they represent the gold standard for rigorous scientific work in the health sciences.

Several writers in prestigious health sciences journals have been observed to advocate for the application of qualitative data to strengthen experimental evidence (Malterud 2001), to assist in the interpretation of the intervention results (Donovan et al. 2002), to explore the relevance of results to patients and improve measures (Gibson et al. 2004) and to move away from an 'either–or' approach to methods (Wallen and Berger 2004: 404). Although advocacy for incorporating qualitative methods into experimental trials has been well documented, these calls provided little insight into the procedures for incorporating the methods. As such a framework was needed for designing such studies and guiding the practice of embedding qualitative data into intervention trials.

A framework for mixed methods intervention trials

The work of Sandelowski (1996) provides a brief framework for thinking about incorporating qualitative methods into experimental intervention studies. She described how 'qualitative methods may be used as components of case, small sample, and larger clinical trials of interventions, before a clinical trial is begun (in studies designed to "trial" the trial) or after a clinical trial is complete' (Sandelowski 1996: 361).

Sandelowski (1996) then suggested that qualitative data could flow into an intervention trial and be used by researchers in three places in the process of the experiment. Figure 9.2 presents a visual interpretation of these ideas for three types of mixed methods embedded intervention designs.

The before-trial design involves collecting and analysing qualitative data before an intervention trial in order to enhance the quality of the subsequent trial. The during-trial design incorporates qualitative data collection into the study during the experiment, while the after-trial design involves collecting and analysing qualitative data as a follow-up to the clinical trial. The purpose of the qualitative data collection is dependent upon when it is collected. Sandelowski (1996) identified

- The **before-trial** mixed methods intervention design: collect qualitative data prior to the trial

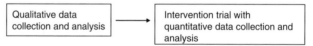

- The **during-trial** mixed methods intervention design: collect qualitative data during the trial

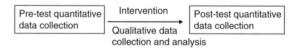

- The **after-trial** mixed methods intervention design: collect qualitative data after the trial

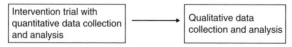

Figure 9.2 Designs for mixed methods intervention trials.

several purposes, including to help determine the best approach for recruiting trial participants, to obtain information about the feasibility and burden the intervention may impose on patients and caregivers, to refine interventions for subsequent trials, to expand the interpretation of the quantitative results to understand why outcomes did or did not occur and to examine more closely individual variation in specific settings. Creswell et al. (2006) listed additional possibilities using the framework of before-, during-, and after-intervention trials as shown in Table 9.1. Because qualitative data are gathered in the field, they add

Table 9.1 Reasons for including qualitative data collection in an intervention trial (adapted from Creswell et al. 2006).

Qualitative data are collected before an intervention trial:

- To develop an instrument for use in intervention trial (when a suitable instrument is not available)
- To develop good recruiting/consent practices for participants into an intervention trial
- To understand the participants, context and environment so that an intervention would work (i.e. applying interventions to real-life situations)
- To document a need for the intervention
- To compile a comprehensive assessment of baseline information

Qualitative data are collected during an intervention trial:

- To validate the quantitative outcomes with qualitative data representing the voices of the participants
- To understand the impact of the intervention on participants (for example, barriers/facilitators)
- To understand unanticipated participant experiences during the trial
- To identify key constructs that might potentially impact the outcomes of the trial, such as changes in the sociocultural environment
- To identify resources that can facilitate the conduct of the intervention
- To understand and depict processes experienced by the experimental groups
- To check the fidelity of the implementation of procedures
- To identify potential mediating and moderating factors

Qualitative data are collected after an intervention trial:

- To understand how participants view the results of the trial
- To receive participant feedback to revise the treatment
- To help explain the quantitative outcomes, such as under-represented variations in the trial outcomes
- To determine the long-term, sustained effects of an intervention after a trial
- To understand in more depth how the mechanisms worked in a theoretical model
- To determine if the processes in conducting the trial had treatment fidelity
- To assess the context when comparisons of outcomes are made with baseline data

'real-life' examples to trials, and because they present individual stories, they provide evocative and compelling ways to communicate the impact of clinical trials to diverse, practitioner audiences. In these ways, qualitative data might enhance some of the limitations inherent in traditional quantitative experiments, such as the report of non-significant results, a focus on group variation at the expense of individual variation, use of inadequate measures, treatment fidelity problems, or challenges in the recruitment and consent of participants.

To illustrate how the embedding of a qualitative data collection might work in practice, Sandelowski (1996) chose the after-trial design to discuss. She described how qualitative data can help explain within- and between-subject variations in outcomes on instruments, verify individual scores on outcomes measures and note discrepancies between the planned intervention and its actual approach.

Despite the conceptual allure of Sandelowski's (1996) framework, it did not have much visibility within the health science literature. One conclusion is that perhaps Sandelowski's (1996) ideas were ahead of her time. In a Science Citation Index (SCI) search of references for her 1996 paper, only 20 citations were found. Of these citations, 17 were in nursing journals or journals edited by nurse researchers and only three were published outside of nursing. Why was her framework not more widely cited across the health sciences? We can only surmise, but we do know that at the time of her publication, conceptualisation of mixed methods designs was an emerging topic in the health sciences literature (Crabtree and Miller 1992), and that a comprehensive set of design-types was not yet published (Creswell et al. 2003; Tashakkori and Teddlie 2003). A notation system for drawing a visual diagram of the procedures was available (Morse 1991), but detailed use of this notation system did not emerge until somewhat later (Creswell et al. 2003). Major books and chapters had yet to be written about mixed methods approaches (Tashakkori and Teddlie 1998, 2003; Creswell 2007). The calls for the implementation of mixed methods intervention studies have come to real prominence only within the last few years (for example, Malterud 2001) and perhaps most importantly, few published studies by 1996 had exhibited models of intervention trials with nested or embedded qualitative data.

Examples of qualitative data in intervention trials

As shown in Tables 9.2–9.4, the topics addressed in the eight studies represent a range of disease issues and different time periods in which the researchers introduced qualitative data (before, during and after the trial). In all eight studies, the qualitative arm played a secondary

Table 9.2 Published examples of before-trial design.

	Donovan et al. (2002)	Brett et al. (2002)
Topic	Prostate testing for cancer and treatment for men	Physical activity and diet for individuals and families in one community
Study aim	A randomised controlled trial (RCT) of two treatments for prostate cancer (with and without monitoring)	A three-phase ethnographic study that explored the factors that affect people's decision about physical activity and diet
Qualitative data collection	In-depth interviews of men after receiving results of prostate test before randomisation	21 open-ended interviews, 12 semi-structured interviews and 6 observations at home with parents with small children
Mixed methods approach	Collected qualitative interview data before RCT to enhance the rate of consent to participation in the trial	Collected ethnographic data to help inform and design the intervention procedures

Table 9.3 Published examples of during-trial design.

	Baskerville et al. (2001)	Victor et al. (2004)	Whittemore et al. (2000)
Topic	Prevention practices implementation guidelines	Self-management and patient education programmes for osteoarthritis (OA)	Social support by peer advisors and myocardial infarction
Study aim	An evaluation study of 22 intervention practices for implementing prevention guidelines by 54 family physicians in Canada	An RCT of health promotion intervention for OA of the knee	Part of an RCT study that explored the experience of providing social support from the perspective of a peer advisor who experienced a myocardial infarction
Qualitative data collection	Monthly narrative reports; telephone interviews; interviews at end of intervention	Open-ended questions, diaries from intervention group and audio-taped education sessions	Peer informants' logs, focused interviews and individual phone interviews
Mixed methods approach	Collected qualitative data and compared it with close-ended questions about physician satisfaction with the intervention	Collected qualitative data during the intervention to converge with data about knowledge of OA and its management, outcomes for treatment and quality of services	Collected qualitative data during the trial and analysed it for themes from peer advisors

Table 9.4 Published examples of after-trial design.

	Snowdon et al. (1998)	Campbell et al. (2001)	Rogers et al. (2003)
Topic	Ventilatory support for critically ill neonates with acute respiratory failure	Reasons for compliance with a home-based exercise regimen by patients with osteoarthritis (OA)	Patient adherence to anti-psychotic medication
Study aim	An RCT of two methods of ventilatory support for critically ill neonates with acute respiratory failure	An RCT of physiotherapy and control interventions in patients with OA of the knee	An RCT of two interventions to improve management of anti-psychotic medication
Qualitative data collection	Interviews with parents in home and by telephone	20 in-depth interviews with intervention participants 5 months and 1 year after intervention	43 in-depth interviews with 16 patients over course of trial
Mixed methods approach	Collected parents' interviews about the content of the results, the level of information presented and their reactions to results after they received the quantitative results	Collected interview qualitative data from patients 3 months and 1 year after the intervention to describe why they did or did not comply with the physiotherapy	Collected qualitative data before the intervention to help construct the intervention; collected data after the trial to develop patient narratives from individuals who had positive scores on the outcome measures

role to the larger intervention trial. The authors called these studies 'nested' studies or 'embedded' studies of qualitative data within randomised controlled trials (for example, Donovan et al. 2002). Different forms of qualitative data were collected, including interviews, observations, narrative reports, focus groups and diaries. The use of qualitative research in these studies was limited to qualitative data collection, instead of the larger framework of qualitative methodology that encompasses philosophical assumptions, the specification of a 'type' of qualitative design such as a case study or grounded theory design, and qualitative interpretations based on the self-reflexivity of the researcher (see Creswell 2007; Denzin and Lincoln 2005). One article, however, did report a complete ethnographic design (Brett et al. 2002).

The reasons for collecting qualitative data related to the timing for the collection of qualitative data, and included: to improve recruitment and consent of participants before the trial (Rogers et al. 2003); to identify barriers and facilitators that could be used in the intervention before the trial (Brett et al. 2002); to compare results from the quantitative data with the qualitative findings (Victor et al. 2004); to evaluate the fidelity of implementing the intervention and how it worked (Baskerville et al. 2001); to gain more detail about the intervention (Whittemore et al. 2000); to follow up on intervention results (Rogers et al. 2003); to obtain feedback from participants to trial results (Snowdon et al. 1998); and to follow up with participants on compliance with an intervention (Campbell et al. 2001). Further, in all of these eight studies, the journal publications reviewed presented only the qualitative data component; the intervention trial was reported in a separate study, a recommended approach to publishing mixed methods studies in family medicine (Stange et al. 2006) (see also Chapter 8). It is also important to note that these were large-scale funded projects, published in international journals between 1998 and 2003.

Several issues surfaced that were related to the specific types of designs. First, in all of the designs, what rationale should be presented by researchers as to why the qualitative data were needed? In Donovan et al. (2002) the interview data were used to help recruit participants to the trial, while in Brett et al. (2002) the intent was to gather ethnographic data to help inform the treatment. Second, both of these studies raised the question as to what specific qualitative information might be useful for enhancing the intervention (for example, answers to questions, themes, general patterns). In a during-trial design, how will the researchers compare the quantitative data with the qualitative data? In Victor et al. (2004), baseline quantitative data were compared with the qualitative data collected during the experiment. The researchers also made comparisons on questions for which they had comparable data for both the quantitative and the qualitative arms. In their study, Baskerville et al. (2001) transformed their qualitative data into counts so that they could be easily compared with the quantitative data. Third, the researchers for during-trial designs were concerned about the qualitative data collection biasing the treatment outcomes. Thus, collecting data at the baseline prior to the experiment or at the 'exit' stage, such as through unobtrusive diaries turned in after the trial, were popular approaches (Baskerville et al. 2001). Fourth, these studies showed collecting qualitative data at different times and at multiple points in the trial (Rogers et al. 2003). Fifth, for after-trial designs, the issue of what cases to select for follow-up surfaced. One study used positive and negative scores on the major outcome variable in the trial as a basis for selecting cases (Rogers et al. 2003). Another study selected individuals from both the treatment and control groups in the trial who had experienced positive outcomes of the trial (Snowdon et al. 1998) and a third study chose only individuals from the intervention arm of the trial (Campbell et al. 2001).

Three illustrative studies

In order to better understand the different stages in the process of intervention research in which the qualitative data entered the trial, three examples were drawn from the eight studies to highlight the possibilities (Donovan et al. 2002; Rogers et al. 2003; Victor et al. 2004). Figures 9.3, 9.4 and 9.5 provide pictorial representations of the processes used in these studies. These diagrams follow the guidelines the authors published for developing these representations (Creswell and Plano Clark 2006) and illustrate the general procedures in boxes. The use of 'qual' in small letters denotes a secondary role for qualitative research, and the use of 'QUAN' in capital letters designates a primary role for quantitative research. In addition, below the large boxes are the specific data collection and analysis procedures undertaken by the researchers. The use of pictorial representations can help make complex data collection and analysis procedures of mixed methods research clearer to the reader.

Donovan et al. (2002) (Figure 9.3) illustrated the before-trial design in which the authors gathered qualitative interview data at the recruitment phase prior to the trial. They used the qualitative data to help them revise the study information, to present the non-radical arm of the study to participants and to make decisions about the best procedures for recruiting participants to the trial. Victor et al. (2004) (Figure 9.4) on the other hand, represented a during-trial collection of qualitative data. During the trial, the researchers asked participants to make entries in diaries. In addition, they tape recorded and subsequently analysed the intervention sessions. In the studies published by Victor et al. (2004) and Donovan et al. (2002), the authors gathered qualitative data and compared them at the end of the trial with quantitative outcomes. In an after-trial qualitative data collection, Rogers et al. (2003) (Figure 9.5) followed up on selected participants who scored positively and negatively on the major outcome measure in order to assess the effectiveness of the intervention in a randomised controlled trial.

Discussion and implications for practice

This discussion has highlighted the potential benefits of adding qualitative data to intervention trials – using a mixed methods intervention

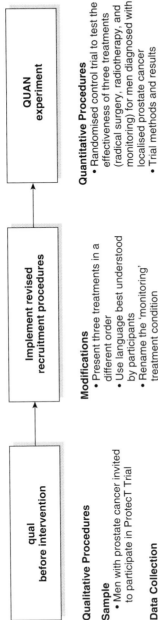

Figure 9.3 Before-intervention mixed methods design (Donovan et al. 2002). Reprinted from Plano Clark, V.L. & Creswell, J.W. (2008). *The Mixed Methods Reader*. Sage Publications, Thousand Oaks, California, with permission of Sage Publications.

---

qual before intervention

Qualitative Procedures

Sample
• Men with prostate cancer invited to participate in ProtecT Trial

Data Collection
• Semistructured interviews
• Audiotapes of recruitment sessions
• Elaboration follow-up interviews with some patients and recruiters about audiotaped sessions

Data Analysis
• Transcription
• Analysed for themes

Findings
• Identified four ways in which the study information was having a negative impact on recruitment

---

Implement revised recruitment procedures

Modifications
• Present three treatments in a different order
• Use language best understood by participants
• Rename the 'monitoring' treatment condition
• Clarity presentation of randomisation and clinical equipoise

Result of Changes
• Increased rate of consent to randomisation from 30%–40% to 70%

QUAN experiment

Quantitative Procedures
• Randomised control trial to test the effectiveness of three treatments (radical surgery, radiotherapy, and monitoring) for men diagnosed with localised prostate cancer
• Trial methods and results reported elsewhere

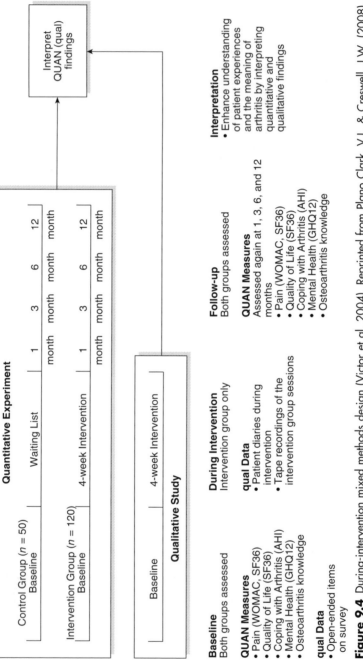

Figure 9.4 During-intervention mixed methods design (Victor et al. 2004). Reprinted from Plano Clark, V.L. & Creswell, J.W. (2008). *The Mixed Methods Reader.* Sage Publications, Thousand Oaks, California, with permission of Sage Publications.

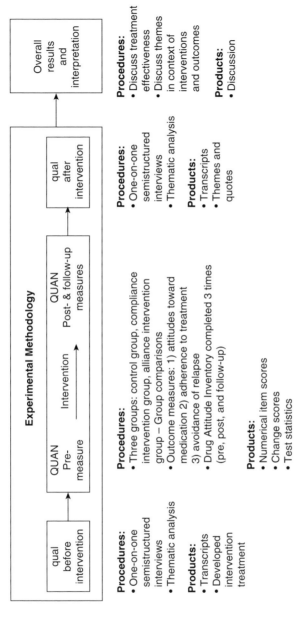

Experimental Methodology

qual before intervention

QUAN Pre-measure

Intervention

QUAN Post- & follow-up measures

qual after intervention

Overall results and interpretation

Procedures:
• One-on-one semistructured interviews
• Thematic analysis

Products:
• Transcripts
• Developed intervention treatment

Procedures:
• Three groups: control group, compliance intervention group, alliance intervention group – Group comparisons
• Outcome measures: 1) attitudes toward medication 2) adherence to treatment 3) avoidance of relapse
• Drug Attitude Inventory completed 3 times (pre, post, and follow-up)

Products:
• Numerical item scores
• Change scores
• Test statistics

Procedures:
• One-on-one semistructured interviews
• Thematic analysis

Products:
• Transcripts
• Themes and quotes

Procedures:
• Discuss treatment effectiveness
• Discuss themes in context of interventions and outcomes

Products:
• Discussion

Figure 9.5 After-intervention mixed methods design (Rogers et al. 2003). Reprinted from Plano Clark, V.L. & Creswell, J.W. (2008). *The Mixed Methods Reader.* Sage Publications, Thousand Oaks, California, with permission of Sage Publications.

design. It also suggests that a systematic analysis of these studies can be made, complete with a focus on the types of qualitative data collected, their use within the intervention framework, their time for inclusion and a visual representation of their use.

There are several implications for practice that emanate from this discussion. First, consideration of the timing (before, during, after) for when qualitative data should be introduced into an intervention trial needs to be driven by the purpose of the data. Second, the researcher needs to be specific about the reasons for incorporating qualitative data into the trial. It is recommended that intervention researchers consider the full list of possible reasons for incorporating qualitative data into their trials and are specific about these reasons in their proposals and reports. Researchers should also consider the potential to use qualitative data at multiple points in the research process, and possible combinations of before-trial, during-trial and after-trial data collection, such as the several points of qualitative data collection illustrated in the study reported by Rogers et al. (2003).

Third, because mixed methods procedures involve multiple forms of data and multiple types of analysis, researchers should include a visual representation of the planned trial to ensure that the reader can follow the research plan. Fourth, the language and philosophy of mixed methods research should be used to guide the trial, rather than simply adding some qualitative data collection to an otherwise quantitative experiment. The language of mixed methods research can help assist individuals who review such projects and need to apply standards for evaluating them (Creswell and Plano Clark 2006). Fifth, when conducting a 'during-trial' procedure, collect the qualitative data on constructs similar to the quantitative data, and enact procedures so that the introduction of the qualitative data collection will not bias the quantitative outcomes. Use of unobtrusive measures such as diaries completed during the experiment and collected at the end of the study will improve controls over treatment bias. For after-trial designs, select individuals that can best provide information about explaining the results. This may mean collecting data from only individuals in the treatment group.

The studies reviewed here are limited to a small number of exemplar studies, and the criteria used to evaluate them have been based on prior components found in social science and primary health care research. It is unknown at this time whether the designs and issues would differ if other forms of experimental designs (for example, quasi- versus randomised controlled trial) or other methods in the health sciences, such as correlational studies, were employed. Further, additional intervention studies with qualitative arms exist beyond those discussed in this paper (for example, Bottorf et al. 2004; Gamel et al. 2001; Hansebo and Kihlgren 2004; Perraud et al. 2004). These additional studies, however, seem to support the three-design framework reported in this chapter.

This review of the literature illustrates that investigations embedding qualitative data within intervention trials are being published, and that a framework of before-, during- and after-trial can help researchers conceptualise the type of embedding procedures that they are using. The review also indicates that exemplars can be found that raise issues that researchers need to consider as they develop their own nested experimental studies. The framework of including qualitative data before-, during-, or after-trial provides a useful model to consider when planning the addition of qualitative data. This chapter further provides a language for discussing the use of qualitative data within intervention trials and begins to raise questions about potential issues that might emerge. The discussion does not exhaustively review the many intervention trials that have incorporated qualitative data, it has utilised models primarily developed in the social sciences and it highlights the need for additional study of issues that need to be anticipated when introducing qualitative data into intervention studies. Despite these limitations, mixed methods research is being conducted in the health sciences and a framework for considering when and why qualitative research is incorporated in these studies is useful information for clinicians. Such a discussion will ultimately advance the understanding of mixed methods in the health sciences.

References

Baskerville N.B., Hogg W. and Lemelin J. (2001) Process evaluation of a tailored multifaceted approach to changing family physician practice patterns and improving preventive care. *Journal of Family Practice*, **50**, 242–249.

Borkan J.M. (2004) Mixed methods studies: a foundation for primary care research. *Annals of Family Medicine*, **2**, 4–6.

Bottorff J.L., Johnson J.L., Moffat B., Fofonoff D., Budz B. and Groening M. (2004) Synchronizing clinician engagement and client motivation in telephone counseling. *Qualitative Health Research*, **14**, 462–477.

Brett J.A., Heimendinger J., Boender C., Morin C. and Marshall J.A. (2002) Using ethnography to improve intervention design. *Journal of Health Promotion*, **16**, 331–340.

Campbell R., Evans M., Tucker M., Quilty B., Pieppe P. and Donovan J.L. (2001) Why don't patients do their exercises: understanding non-compliance with physiotherapy in patients with osteoarthritis of the knee. *Journal of Epidemiological Community Health*, **55**, 132–138.

Crabtree B.F. and Miller W.L. (1992) *Doing Qualitative Research*. Newbury Park, CA: Sage Publications.

Creswell J.W. (2007) *Qualitative Inquiry and Research Design: Choosing Among Five Approaches*. Thousand Oaks, California: Sage Publications.

Creswell J.W. (2008) *Educational Research: Planning, Conducting, and Evaluating Quantitative and Qualitative Research*. Upper Saddle River, New Jersey: Pearson Merrill Prentice Hall.

Creswell J.W. and Plano Clark V. (2006) *Designing and Conducting Mixed Methods Research*. Thousand Oaks, California: Sage Publications.

Creswell J.W., Fetters M.D. and Ivankova N.V. (2004) Designing a mixed methods study in primary care. *Annals of Family Medicine*, **2**, 7–12.

Creswell J.W., Plano Clark V.L., Gutmann M.L. and Hanson W.E. (2003) Advanced mixed methods research designs. In Tashakkori A. and Teddlie C. (eds.) *Handbook of Mixed Methods in Social and Behavioral Research*, pp. 209–240. Thousand Oaks, California: Sage Publications.

Creswell J.W., Shope R., Plano Clark V.L. and Green D.O. (2006) How interpretive qualitative research extends mixed methods research. *Research in the Schools*, **13**, 1–11.

Denzin N.K. and Lincoln Y.S. (2005) *The Sage Handbook of Qualitative Research*. Thousand Oaks, California: Sage Publications.

Donovan J., Mills N., Smith M., Brindle L., Jacoby A. and Peters T. (2002) Improving design and conduct of randomized trials by embedding them in qualitative research: ProtecT (prostate testing for cancer and treatment) study. *British Medical Journal*, **325**, 766–769.

Eliot J. (2005) *Using Narrative in Social Research: Qualitative and Quantitative Approaches*. London: Sage Publications.

Gamel C., Grypdonck M., Hengeveld M. and Davis B. (2001) A method to develop a nursing intervention: the contribution of qualitative studies to the process. *Journal of Advanced Nursing*, **33**, 806–819.

Giacomini M.K. and Cook D.J. (2000) Users' guides to the medical literature: XXIII. Qualitative research in health care. A. Are the results valid? *Journal of the American Medical Association*, **284**, 357–362.

Gibson G., Timlin A., Curran S. and Wattis J. (2004) The scope for qualitative methods in research and clinical trials in dementia. *Age and Aging*, **33**, 422–426.

Greene J.C. and Caracelli V.J. (eds.) (1997) *Advances in Mixed-Method Evaluation: The Challenges and Benefits of Integrating Diverse Paradigms* (New Directions for Evaluation, No. 74). San Francisco: Jossey-Bass.

Hansebo G. and Kihlgren M. (2004) Nursing home care: changes after supervision. *Journal of Advanced Nursing*, **45**, 269–279.

Hanson W.E., Creswell J.W., Plano Clark V.L. and Petska K.S. (2005) Mixed methods research in counseling psychology. *Journal of Counseling Psychology*, **52**, 1–12.

Harrison A. (2007) *A longitudinal, embedded, sequential design of a teacher education mentoring program*. Unpublished dissertation, University of Nebraska.

Howe K.R. (2004) A critique of experimentalism. *Qualitative Inquiry*, **10**, 42–61.

Kutner J.S., Steiner J.F., Corbett K.K., Jahnigen D.W. and Barton P.L. (1999) Information needs in terminal illness. *Social Science Medicine*, **48**, 1341–1352.

Luck L., Jackson D. and Usher K. (2006) Case study: a bridge across the paradigms. *Nursing Inquiry*, **13**, 103–109.

Malterud K. (2001) The art and science of clinical knowledge: evidence beyond measures and numbers. *Lancet*, **358**, 397–400.

Marvel M.K., Staehling S. and Henricks B. (1991) A taxonomy of clinical research methods: comparisons of family practice and general medical journals. *Family Medicine*, **23**, 202–207.

McIlvain H.E., Backer E.L., Crabtree B.F. and Lacy N. (2002) Physician attitudes and the use of office-based activities for tobacco control. *Family Medicine*, **34**, 114–119.

McVea K., Crabtree B.F. and Medder J.D. (1996) An ounce of prevention? Evaluation of 'Put Prevention into Practice' program. *Journal of Family Practice*, **43**, 361–369.

Morse J.M. (1991) Approaches to qualitative–quantitative methodological triangulation. *Nursing Research*, **40**, 120–123.

National Institutes of Health (1999) *Qualitative Methods in Health Research: Opportunities and Considerations in Application and Review*. Washington, D.C.: National Institutes of Health.

Nutting P.A., Rost K., Dickinson M., Werner J.J., Dickinson P., Smith J.L. et al. (2002) Barriers to initiating depression treatment in primary care practice. *Journal of General Internal Medicine*, **17**, 103–111.

Perraud S., Farran C.J., Loukissa D. and Paun O. (2004) Alzheimer's disease caregiving information and skills, part III: Group. *Research in Nursing and Health*, **27**, 110–120.

Plano Clark V.L. (2005) Cross-disciplinary analysis of the use of mixed methods in physics education research, counseling psychology, and primary care. PhD dissertation. The University of Nebraska-Lincoln, USA. Retrieved September 30, 2008, from Dissertations & Theses: A & I database. (Publication No. AAT 3163998.)

Plano Clark V. and Creswell J.W. (2008) *The Mixed Methods Reader*. Thousand Oaks, California: Sage Publications.

Rogers A., Day J., Randall F. and Bentall R.P. (2003) Patients' understanding and participation in a trial designed to improve the management of anti-psychotic medication. *Social Psychiatry Psychiatric Epidemiology*, **38**, 720–727.

Sandelowski M. (1996) Using qualitative methods in intervention studies. *Research in Nursing and Health*, **19**, 359–364.

Snowdon C., Garcia J. and Elbourne D. (1998) Reactions of participants to the results of a randomised controlled trial: exploratory study. *British Medical Journal*, **317**, 21–26.

Stange K.C., Crabtree B.F. and Miller W.L. (2006) Publishing multimethod research. *Annals of Family Medicine*, **4**, 292–294.

Tashakkori A. and Teddlie C. (1998) *Mixed Methodology: Combining Qualitative and Quantitative Approaches.* Thousand Oaks, California: Sage Publications.

Tashakkori A. and Teddlie C. (eds.) (2003) *Handbook of Mixed Methods in Social and Behavioral Research.* Thousand Oaks, California: Sage Publications.

Victor C.R., Ross F. and Axford J. (2004) Capturing lay perspectives in a randomized control trial of a health promotion intervention for people with osteoarthritis of the knee. *Journal of Evaluation in Clinical Practice,* **10**, 63–70.

Wallen G.R. and Berger A. (2004) Mixed methods: In search of truth in palliative care medicine. *Journal of Palliative Medicine,* **7**, 403–404.

Whittemore R., Rankin S.H., Callahan C.D., Leder M.C. and Carroll D.L. (2000) The peer advisor experience providing social support. *Qualitative Health Research,* **10**(2), 260–276.

A Mixed Methods Sequential Explanatory Study: Police Referrals to a Psychiatric Facility

Reshin Maharaj, Sharon Andrew, Louise O'Brien and Donna Gillies

Introduction

This aim of this chapter is to provide the reader with a 'real-life' example of the development and application of a sequential explanatory design. The project that is described is a doctoral study which examined police referrals to a psychiatric facility. The quantitative aspect of the study sought to investigate the characteristics of persons referred by the police to a mental facility, whilst the qualitative aspect explored the experiences of nurses caring for patients referred by the police. This chapter will outline the design considerations as well as describing aspects of the study to highlight the practical challenges faced in conducting mixed methods research as part of a doctoral programme.

The project

Police have become a major source of referrals to psychiatric services and this practice has changed the profile of patients admitted to these services. Individuals referred to psychiatric services by police, however, may not necessarily be those who will benefit from hospitalisation. A change in the patient profile of a psychiatric facility may have a major impact for mental health nursing and the centrality of the therapeutic interpersonal nurse–patient relationship.

This project explored police referrals to a psychiatric facility. The focus in the quantitative first phase was the differences in the demographic, diagnostic and admission outcomes, for police referrals and referrals from other sources. This phase involved an audit of the medical records for 200 patients admitted to a psychiatric facility during a 6-month period. The second phase was conducted utilising a Heideggerian phenomenological framework to explore the nurses' experiences of caring for patients referred by the police (Heiddeger 1962, 2005 – translated by Dhalstrom). Nine nurses working in three acute units of a psychiatric hospital were interviewed in this phase. The qualitative data expanded upon and enhanced the understanding of the nurses' experiences of police referrals to a psychiatric facility.

Background

The 1970s witnessed major changes to the care of people with chronic mental illness in Australia (Happell 2005). Australian mental health care had moved from custodial asylumdom to community-centred care (NSW Mental Health Sentinel Events Review Committee 2003). The result was a reduction in the number of hospital beds and an increase in the number of people with chronic mental health problems in communities who otherwise would be in psychiatric hospitals (Pogrebin and Poole 1987; NSW Mental Health Sentinel Events Review Committee 2003). Assertive policies of deinstitutionalisation were being implemented in most developed countries internationally (Happell 2007). The policy positioned the acute hospital to be utilised for acute care only, with preventive measures and rehabilitation taking place in the community (Select Committee on Mental Health 2002). The aim of deinstitutionalisation was to provide an opportunity for better treatment and improved life chances for people with mental illness (Happell 2007).

As the number of patients in psychiatric hospitals decreased, police contact with people with a mental illness increased. Studies conducted in the US indicated that in the absence of sufficient community support, those with mental illness posed a variety of problems for local communities and often became the object of citizen complaints to the police (Pogrebin and Poole 1987). Although law enforcement agencies have always had a long history of community intervention with persons with mental illness, the intensity of their involvement altered as more patients with mental health problems were released into the community (Select Committee on Mental Health 2002). Due to the mass exodus of psychiatric patients into the community setting, police became increasingly the first to respond to crisis calls and have become a first line of contact for people who are mentally disturbed (Meadows et al. 1994; NSW Health 1998; Fry et al. 2002; McCann and Clark 2003; Boyd 2006; Lee 2006). Studies in the US, UK and Australia indicate that police departments have become the most utilised agencies for psychiatric referral (Dunn and Fahey 1987; Pogrebin and Poole 1987; Meadows et al. 1994; Select Committee on Mental Health 2002).

In New South Wales, Australia, while the police were not formally trained to recognise and assess mental illness, they have statutory authority to take persons whom they perceive to be mentally ill into custody for emergency examination and hospitalisation (Boyd and Semmler 2006). Much of the knowledge and skills police demonstrate in dealing with the mentally ill are acquired through on-the-job experience, and Fry et al. (2002) report that an attitude prevailed within the police culture that dealing with mentally disturbed people was not considered 'real police work'.

Although recent Australian studies have addressed police referrals of patients to emergency departments (Lee 2006; Fisher 2007), few Australian studies have addressed referrals made by police to psychiatric services (Meadows et al. 1994; Kneebone et al. 1995). Findings from the two previously published studies of police referrals indicated that: 1) the rates of major mental illnesses such as the schizophrenias and the affective disorders of mania and depression were much lower in comparison to the rates in the US and the UK; 2) persons with substance misuse and persons who threatened self-harm or suicide were a high indicator for police referrals; and 3) non-psychotic subjects referred by police suffered mostly from severe personality disorders and presented major management difficulties for staff, consequently increasing the risk of the medicalisation of criminal behaviour (Meadows et al. 1994, Kneebone et al. 1995).

There appear to be clinical differences in patients referred by police compared to those referred by other sources, such as community services, self, family and general practitioner (McNeil et al. 1991; Meadows et al. 1994; Kneebone et al. 1995; Spurrell et al. 2003). These differences are generally in relation to clinical characteristics of patients with studies indicating that patients referred by the police have lower rates of serious mental illnesses or psychotic illness (Meadows et al. 1994; Kneebone et al. 1995; Spurrell et al. 2003), but higher rates of behavioural problems that are complex and challenging in terms of their illness and behaviour in comparison to referrals from other sources (McNeil et al. 1991).

While there are qualitative studies that have explored the role of the nurse in caring for mentally ill patients (Cleary and Edwards 1999; Cutliffe et al. 2005; Shattell et al. 2006), there are few studies that have addressed the implications of police referral for mental health nursing. Moreover, there are few studies that have used a mixed methods approach to this area of nursing research (Higgins et al. 1999; Jenkins and Coffey 2002).

Rationale for a mixed methods approach

Nursing knowledge and practice are increasingly expected to be based on the best available evidence (Flemming 2007). Where that evidence is limited, researchers are challenged to determine the most appropriate approach to acquire the evidence. The depth of insight into the research problem made available by mixed methods research makes it highly suitable for studying many complex nursing and health care research problems. Mixed methods research offers nurses the opportunity to conduct research that is relevant to nurses whilst still providing a rigorous methodological framework (Andrew and Halcomb 2006; Flemming 2007).

Although police represent an important source of referrals under the NSW Mental Health Act (NSW Institute of Psychiatry 1998), few studies have addressed police referrals to psychiatric services either quantitatively or qualitatively or in combination; a doctoral research programme was designed to explore police referrals to a psychiatric facility. A mixed methods approach seemed the best fit for the purpose of this research study because of the complexity of the research problem which called for answers beyond simple numbers in a quantitative sense or words in a qualitative sense.

The purpose of the study

It was decided that investigating the demographic and clinical characteristics of patients referred by the police through comparisons with referrals from other sources was best answered through quantitative research methods, whereas exploring the experiences of nurses caring for patients referred by the police required a qualitative approach. The inclusion of the qualitative data served multiple purposes. Firstly, it could complement the quantitative data by clarifying and thereby explaining some of the results from this method. Secondly, as it was focusing on a related but different area of the problem it could broaden or expand the scope of study.

In this chapter we focus on the issues of drug and alcohol and suicidal behaviour of patients referred by police to a mental health facility including some statistical results and the qualitative theme 'expecting the worst'.

Choosing a research design

In addition to justifying the decision to utilise mixed methods in their doctoral studies the student must be able to justify to the reader, and examiner, why a particular mixed methods research design was chosen. The decision about the nature of mixed methods design chosen for this study was guided by responses to the questions regarding the sequence, priority, theoretical perspective (Creswell and Plano Clark 2007) and the purpose of the research being undertaken (see Chapter 3).

While the research problem may be a primary reason underscoring the choice of a design, the researcher still has an element of choice in the type of design chosen for a study. Creswell and Plano Clark's (2007) description of the four major types of mixed methods design was used as a guide in this decision. The triangulated and explanatory designs were both considered. As the qualitative component of the study was to explain and expand the quantitative data the explanatory design was chosen. The advantages of this design include the fact that the researcher conducts the two methods in two separate phases and collects only one type of data at a time (Creswell and Plano Clark 2007). This was seen to represent a more manageable project within the scope of a doctoral programme. Within the explanatory design there are two variations: the follow-up explanations model and the participant selection model. The difference between the two models lies in the connection of the two phases. For this study, the follow-up explanations model was used to explain or expand on the quantitative results by collecting qualitative data from selected participants who could best help explain these findings.

The sequence

The study was conducted in two sequential phases. The first phase involved the (quantitative) audit of the patient records. These data were collected and analysed prior to the commencement of the qualitative phase. The questions used in the second (qualitative) phase were informed by findings that emerged from the stage one data.

The priority

Although the quantitative data were collected first they were not afforded priority as both data collection methods/phases were given equal status in this study.

Integration

Although the quantitative data were collected first and informed some of the questions for the qualitative data collection, true integration of the results occurred in the discussion chapter. Some integration of the quantitative results occurred in the summary for the qualitative chapter.

Theoretical perspective

The philosophical foundation which formed the worldview for conducting this mixed methods research study centred around pragmatism, which draws on many ideas including 'what works', through the use of diverse approaches and placing value on both objective and subjective knowledge.

Hermeneutics based on the work of Heidegger (1962, 2005) and van Manen (1990) provided a guiding framework for the conduct of the qualitative study as it is concerned with exploring, describing and discovering the lived experiences of subjects in context. Phenomenology 'aims at gaining a deeper understanding of the nature or meaning of our everyday experiences' and asks 'what is this or that kind of experience like?' (van Manen 1990: 9). Phenomenology with its philosophical basis in human experience has become a valued and useful mode of extending nurses' understanding of health and illness. Through utilisation of a framework informed by Heideggerian hermeneutic phenomenology, it was possible to explore the broad question 'What does the experience of caring for persons referred by the police mean to nurses?'

The study aim

The overarching aim that guided this mixed methods study was an exploration of police referrals to a psychiatric facility. Specific aims were also developed to guide the separate qualitative and quantitative phases of the study.

The aim of the quantitative phase was to compare the demographic characteristics, diagnoses, admission outcomes and reasons for admission of patients referred by police to the mental health service to the characteristics of patients referred from other sources.

Hypotheses were developed to guide the quantitative data analysis. An example of one hypothesis was: there will be a difference in the percentage of patients referred by police presenting with drug and alcohol problems compared to patients referred by other sources.

Data collection

The study was undertaken in Sydney, Australia, at a major metropolitan mental health facility. Medical records of the first 100 patients referred by the police and by other sources during a 6-month period were reviewed to collect the quantitative data ($n = 200$). The quantitative analysis consisted of statistically testing the various hypotheses. Qualitative data were gathered through interviews with nine nurses employed in the mental health facility. The analysis of qualitative data involved aggregating words into categories of information and presenting the diversity of ideas gathered during data collection. The qualitative data were categorised into themes informed by the work of van Manen (1990). Ethical approval for the study was obtained from the appropriate Human Research Ethics Committees prior to commencing the study. Pseudonyms are used when reporting interview narrative to maintain participant anonymity.

Phase one: sample quantitative findings

In the 6-month study period a total number of 1462 persons were referred to the hospital and evaluated by the admitting duty medical officer. This included 269 persons referred by police and 1193 persons referred by 'other sources' (community mental health teams; hospitals outside the area health service; hospitals within the area health service; self referrals; families/relatives; mental health facilities; psychiatrists/GPs; psychologists/welfare workers). Although not all persons referred to hospital are admitted, the percentage of persons admitted to the hospital from both sources was very similar with 54% ($n = 146$) of patients referred by the police and 51% ($n = 609$) of those referred by other sources. An audit of 200 patients' medical records was undertaken with the first 100 patients from each group (police and other) selected for analysis. Given the constraints of the chapter, the results for substance misuse and suicidality are the only quantitative results presented as an exemplar.

Hypothesis: there will be a difference in the percentage of patients referred by police presenting with drug and alcohol problems compared to patients referred by other sources.

Result: there was a significantly higher proportion of patients presenting with drug and alcohol problems in the police referred group ($n = 72$, 71%) compared to the patients referred by other sources ($n = 49$, 50%: $\chi^2 = 9.94$, d.f. $= 1$, $P = 0.00$). This included patients with a primary diagnosis of substance misuse as well as patients presenting with a secondary diagnosis of substance misuse. This hypothesis was therefore accepted.

Hypothesis: there will be a difference in the percentage of patients referred by police presenting with suicidal behaviour compared to patients referred by other sources.

Result: there was no significant difference between the percentage of patients presenting with suicidal behaviour ($n = 29$, 29%) in the police referred group compared to the patients referred by other sources ($n = 20$, 20%: $\chi^2 = 1.96$, d.f. $= 1$, $P = 0.16$). This hypothesis was therefore rejected.

Phase two: examples of qualitative findings

Nine nurses employed at the psychiatric facility were interviewed. The average length of each interview was 1 hour. The interviews were audio-recorded and transcribed verbatim. The transcripts were then analysed according to phenomenological methods (van Manen 1990). One theme was labelled 'expecting the worst' from police. The sub-themes and their content areas are given in Table 10.1. Under the theme 'expecting the worst', nurse participants described the clinical and diagnostic characteristics of patients referred by the police and explained why some patients were regarded as 'the worst'. Nurses also discussed in detail some of the measures implemented to reduce or eliminate the potential of violence amongst certain patients, in an effort to ensure the safety of the patients and others. This chapter presents the findings for the subtheme 'Being judgemental about patients' as an exemplar.

Table 10.1 Subthemes and subcategories for the theme 'expecting the worst'.

Subtheme	Subcategories
Being judgemental about patients	• They mainly abuse substances • Are they like 'normal referrals'? • Are they suicidal?
Making safety a priority	• Hoping for a response to treatment • Medicating for safety • Secluding for safety

The subtheme 'being judgemental about patients' was concerned with the preconceptions that nurses have about patients that have been referred to a mental health facility by the police. When alerted to the admission of patients referred by police, nurse participants anticipated the arrival of the 'worst' patients. The 'worst' patients often referred to those who abused either illicit substances and/or alcohol which resulted in aggressive or unpredictable behavioural problems. As David explained:

> I suppose from experience we expect the worst [from police referrals] but that's not always the case. I mean you get quite a variety of patients that come through, some extremely agitated and hostile, some quite placid and cooperative and seemingly understanding the process that takes place and cooperating with it . . . Sometimes we seem to have more people with mood disorders and then more people with drug-induced psychosis and/or people with more aggression than before . . . So they're not always aggressive . . . but of all the aggressive patients the police would probably bring in the most extreme . . . and I suppose if there is any wrong aspect . . . it seems to be the drug nature of the patients . . .

There was agreement amongst participants that the majority of patients referred by the police were likely to be affected by illicit substances. As the experience of participants was that these patients were reportedly more likely to be behaviourally disturbed, this may be why they expect the worst of these patients. Wayne, for example, said 'usually the ones that the police bring in are the ones who are the most disturbed . . . probably 9 times out of 10 it is drug induced'. Wayne described the disturbed behaviour displayed by some of the patients who misused substances: '. . . they are so wound up . . . they've gone right to crisis point . . . all they want to do is fight, they are not coherent, they are irrational, they are agitated, they are often very delusional . . .'

In addition to illicit drugs, participants anticipated that patients referred by the police would also have problems with alcohol: 'When there's substances [illicit] . . . there's drugs and alcohol involved' (Terrence). Moreover this combination compounds the influence on these persons' behaviour including their risk of suicide:

> Virtually they are coming in here to sleep it off because inevitably the alcohol depresses them, they have too much of it and then all their troubles brim over and they want to kill themselves so the police bring them here because they are a safety risk. One of the criteria for coming to the hospital is to be a suicide risk. (Janet)

Nurses have expectations of what they consider to be 'normal referrals' to a mental health facility such as patients who presented with symptoms of a major mental illness. Police referrals are judged against these expectations.

> . . . Like I said earlier . . . on those occasions that police bring patients in and they come in . . . they're actually quite like a normal referral, from the community or wherever . . . and those cases are . . . actually a lot of them are chronic schizophrenia . . . on presentation there is every evidence of persecutory ideas and paranoia and all that . . . Police probably have happened to pick them up in the street or something and bring them in. These are the cases that when they arrive they are just like any other normal presentation that we have, and they are brought in by police . . . and then we are able to assess – 'oh yeah, their symptoms does not pose a risk to us, they don't require confinement at that stage. (Lily)

Participants described mixed experiences and feelings about police referrals of suicidal patients. On one hand participants recognised that failure to admit to hospital a person at risk of suicide may lead to undesired outcomes, but on the other hand there was scepticism that some persons were exploiting police to avoid a criminal charge or to exploit the health system by seeking a bed for the night. Eddie said for example that some patients were 'using the mental health system' and were benefiting from their admission to the hospital:

> '. . . like they know that the hospital is safe, it's free . . . they don't have to spend money, they have a clean bed, a roof over their head, they don't have to do anything, they don't have to shower, to wash . . . and they can be here and have the attention'.

Discussion

The interview findings for the sequential explanatory mixed methods research design undertaken, as anticipated, provided explanation and expansion to the quantitative findings. Integration of the datasets was undertaken by developing matrixes (Miles and Huberman 1994). An example of one of these matrices is presented in Table 10.2. As Table 10.2 demonstrates, there was confirmation between the quantitative and qualitative findings in relation to patients referred by police tending to be more likely affected by illicit drugs and/or alcohol than those referred by other sources. The qualitative findings provide expansion in our understanding of what this means to nurses who need to establish a therapeutic relationship with these patients.

Table 10.2 Matrix comparing qualitative and quantitative findings.

Issue	Quantitative findings	Qualitative findings	Integration
Drug and alcohol	Statistically significant difference between police and other referrals	Nurses expect patients referred by police to be on illicit drugs, alcohol Nurses also expect patients' behaviour to be aggressive or unpredictable	Confirmation between two datasets Qualitative findings provide expansion to quantitative findings
Suicide	No statistically significant difference between police and other referrals	Nurses expect patients referred by police to be suicidal Patients referred by the police may be exploiting the health system Nurses make judgements about police referrals against what they expect from 'normal referrals'	Disparity between qualitative and quantitative findings Qualitative findings provided expansion to the quantitative findings Qualitative findings provided expansion to the quantitative findings

The findings also indicate a discrepancy between nurses' expectations about the suicidality of patients referred by the police. The challenge for future research is to seek an understanding of why this is the case. Explanations may include the relatively small quantitative sample size not having sufficient power to detect a small difference between the groups. On the other hand, caring for patients who have been a suicide risk may have had a strong impact on nurses' memories resulting in them linking this back to the fact that the patients were police referrals to the mental health facility.

Nurses' comments provided insight into data that are not available by other means such as: were patients referred by police 'genuinely' mentally ill or are they 'using the system'? The noteworthy finding, however, was that patients who are police referrals are judged against a hypothetical 'normal' patient and 'normal behaviour' for a mental health facility with police referrals seen as being outside this norm and therefore these patients were viewed as the 'worst' until they were assessed as being otherwise. This judgement has an impact on the establishment of a therapeutic relationship with a patient which was revealed in additional qualitative themes.

Conclusion

This mixed methods sequential explanatory design allowed for the exploration of police referrals to a psychiatric facility. In the conduct and design of the study, the qualitative and quantitative data were considered to be of equal significance. The qualitative data were collected and analysed informed by Heideggerian phenomenology. The data generated allowed for a richer and deeper understanding of the research problem than would have been possible from either method of data collection in isolation.

References

Andrew S. and Halcomb E.J. (2006) Mixed methods research is an effective method of enquiry for working with families and communities. *Contemporary Nurse*, **23**, 145–153.

Boyd E. (2006) Appropriate use of *police* officers. *Psychiatric Services*, **57**, 1811.

Boyd R. and Semmler S. (2006) Knowledge of Section 23 of the Mental Health Act. *Australasian Emergency Nursing Journal*, **8**, 149–155.

Cleary M. and Edwards C. (1999) 'Something always comes up': nurse–patient interaction in an acute psychiatric setting. *Journal of Psychiatric and Mental Health Nursing*, **6**, 469–477.

Creswell J.W. and Plano Clark V.L. (2007) *Designing and Conducting Mixed Methods Research*. Thousand Oaks, California: Sage Publications.

Cutliffe J.R., Stevenson C., Jackson S. and Smith P. (2005) A modified grounded theory study of how psychiatric nurses work with suicidal people. *International Journal of Nursing Studies*, **43**, 791–802.

Dunn J. and Fahey T.A. (1987) Section 136 and the police. *Bulletin of the Royal College of Psychiatrists*, **11**, 224–225.

Fisher J.E. (2007) Mental health nurses: de facto police. *International Journal of Mental Health Nursing*, **16**, 230–235.

Flemming K. (2007) The knowledge base for evidence-based nursing. *Advances in Nursing Science*, **30**, 41–51.

Fry A.J., O'Riordan D.P. and Geanellos R. (2002) Social control agents or front-line carers for people with mental health problems: police and mental health services in Sydney, Australia. *Health and Social Care in the Community*, **10**, 277–286.

Happell B. (2005) Mental health nursing: challenging stigma and discrimination towards people experiencing a mental illness. *International Journal of Mental Health Nursing*, **14**, 1.

Happell B. (2007) Appreciating the importance of history: a brief historical overview of mental health, mental health nursing and education in

Australia. *International Journal of Psychiatric Nursing Research*, **12**, 1439–1445.

Heiddeger M. (1962) *Being and Time*. Oxford: Blackwell Publishing.

Heiddeger M. (translated by Dhalstrom D.O.) (2005) *Introduction to Phenomeno-logical Research*. Indiana University Press, Bloomington.

Higgins R., Hurst K. and Wistow G. (1999) Nursing acute psychiatric patients: a quantiative and qualitative study. *Journal of Advanced Nursing*, **29**, 52–63.

Jenkins E. and Coffey M. (2002) Compelled to interact: forensic community mental health nurses' and service users' relationships. *Journal of Psychiatric and Mental Health Nursing*, **9**, 553–562.

Kneebone P., Rogers J. and Hafner J. (1995) Characteristics of police referrals to a psychiatric emergency unit in Australia. *Psychiatric Services*, **46**, 620–622.

Lee S. (2006) The characteristics of police presentations to an emergency department in a community hospital. *Australasian Emergency Nursing Journal*, **9**, 65–72.

van Manen M. (1990) *Researching Lived Experience. Human Science for an Action Sensitive Pedagogy*. Albany, New York: State University of New York Press.

McCann T.V. and Clark E. (2003) A grounded theory study of the role that nurses play in increasing clients' willingness to access community mental health services. *International Journal of Mental Health Nursing*, **12**, 279–288.

McNeil D.E., Hatcher C., Zeiner H., Wolfe H.E. and Myers R.S. (1991) Characteristics of persons referred by the police to the psychiatric emergency room. *Hospital and Community Psychiatry*, **42**, 425–427.

Meadows G., Calder G. and Van Den Bos H. (1994) Police referrals to a psychiatric hospital: Indicators for referral and psychiatric outcome. *Australian and New Zealand Journal of Psychiatry*, **28**, 259–268.

Miles M.B. and Huberman A.M. (1994) *Qualitative Data Analysis: an Expanded Sourcebook*. Thousand Oaks, California: Sage Publications.

NSW Health (1998) *Memorandum of Understanding between NSW Police and NSW Health*. Sydney: NSW Health, NSW Police Service.

NSW Institute of Psychiatry (1998) *Mental Health Act: Guide Book*. Paramatta: NSW Institute of Psychiatry.

NSW Mental Health Sentinel Events Review Committee (2003) *Tracking Tragedy: A Systematic Look at Suicides and Homicides Amongst Mental Health Patients*. Sydney: NSW Health Department.

Pogrebin M. and Poole E. (1987) Deinstitutionalisation and increased arrest rates among the mentally disordered. *Journal of Psychiatry and Law*, Spring, 117–125.

Select Committee on Mental Health (2002) *Inquiry into Mental Health Services in NSW*. NSW Parliament. Legislative Council. Parliamentary Paper No. 368, NSW.

Shattell M.M., McAllister S., Hogan B. and Thomas S.P. (2006) 'She took the time to make sure she understood': mental health patients' experience of being understood. *Archives of Psychiatric Nursing*, **20**, 234–241.

Spurrell M., Hatfield B. and Perry A. (2003) Characteristics of patients presenting for emergency psychiatric assessment at an English hospital. *Psychiatric Services*, **54**, 240–245.

Action Research as a Mixed Methods Design: a Palliative Approach in Residential Aged Care

Jane Phillips and Patricia M. Davidson

Introduction

The philosophical premises of action research and the pragmatic characteristics of mixed methods research are highly congruent. Action research involves the engaging of participants as partners to improve a situation or address an identified problem through cycles of reflection, planning, action and evaluation (Reason and Bradbury 2001). Importantly, action research is a responsive and dynamic process that allows the complex array of predisposing and contributing issues to be considered, impacts of interventions and interactions observed, outcomes noted and action planned (Winter and Munn-Giddings 2001). A range of data collection methods is applicable to action research, including a mixed methods approach due to its applicability to survey, evaluation and field research. A mixed methods approach is particularly useful as it allows multifaceted observations and adaptation of a range of research methodologies to a research setting and questions with unique characteristics (Creswell and Plano Clark 2006).

The aim of this chapter is to provide the reader with a 'real-life' example of the development, implementation and evaluation of an action research project using a mixed methods design. The project that will be described is the Residential–Palliative Approach Competency (R-PAC) Project (Phillips 2007). This project sought to collaboratively develop, implement and evaluate a sustainable model of care to facilitate the delivery of a palliative approach to care for older people admitted to residential aged care facilities, in regional Australia. This chapter will outline the philosophical premises of action research and the mixed methods approach and will use this example to highlight both the theoretical issues and the practical challenges faced in conducting action research in the health sector.

The Residential–Palliative Approach Competency (R-PAC) Project

Despite the common association with cancer, palliative care clinicians are exploring more inclusive and accessible models of care that address contemporary epidemiological trends (Wasson 2000). The trilogy of population ageing, biomedical advances and increasing consumer expectations are challenging the way in which health care is provided to older people in residential aged care (Davies and Higginson 2004). Similar to other parts of the developed world, Australian residential aged care facilities predominantly care for older people who require skilled nursing care, those who are dying and lack a full-time carer, or those whose care needs exceed community resources. This care setting is increasingly becoming the place of death for many older people, with approximately 20% of new residents in Australia dying within 12 months of being admitted to permanent care (Australian Institute of Health and Welfare 2004). In spite of the frequency of death in this setting, the majority of older people dying in residential aged care will have their end-of-life care delivered by doctors, nurses (registered and enrolled nurses) and care assistants (unregulated workers) who are not palliative care specialists.

Previous research has identified numerous obstacles to providing palliative care in residential aged care, including: inadequate staffing levels; a regulatory focus on rehabilitation; staff inexperienced in evidence-based palliative care; failure to recognise treatment futility; lack of communication amongst decision makers, residents and families; and failure to implement a timely end-of-life care plan (Australian Department of Health and Ageing and National Health and Medical Research Council 2006). In Australia, public policy has acknowledged that a palliative approach within residential aged care is required to effectively care for residents whose condition is not amenable to cure, either as a consequence of the ageing process or a specific condition (Australian Department of Health and Ageing and National Health and Medical Research Council 2006). This evidence-based approach to palliative care for older people integrates the key principles of gerontology, geriatrics and palliative care (Currow and Hegarty 2006). The *Guidelines for a Palliative Approach in Residential Aged Care* (Australian Department of Health and Ageing and National Health and Medical

Research Council 2006) set out a new way of appraising and addressing the palliative care needs of older people in residential aged care. Importantly, these guidelines reinforce the need for a palliative approach throughout an older person's residential care trajectory, rather than merely restricting the focus to terminal care.

The R-PAC Project, used as an exemplar of action research in this book, was designed to address the unmet needs of people requiring palliative care services in residential aged care in a regional Australian community setting. We adopted a mixed methods design because of the conceptual and methodological congruence with the study aims.

Reconciling mixed methods research in an action research paradigm

The residential aged care setting is a complex health care environment that is characterised by stringent regulatory requirements (Commonwealth Department of Health and Aged Care 1997), a heterogeneous workforce and a need for multidisciplinary care (Royal Australian College of General Practitioners 2006). Residents in this setting are becoming older, increasingly frail, presenting with multiple co-morbidities, have high care needs and are likely to have some degree of cognitive impairment challenging contemporary care models (Phillips et al. 2006a). The predominant care providers in this setting are care assistants, who have little or no formal training and are supervised by a smaller number of registered nurses (Commonwealth Department of Health and Aged Care 1997). Developing a sustainable model for the delivery of a palliative approach for older people in residential aged care required an in-depth understanding of the human activities and systems operating in this dynamic health care setting.

Explorations of a range of epistemological and epidemiological frameworks guided the R-PAC Project. Action research, with its focus on improving and involving, was considered to be the methodology most likely to engage residential aged care providers in a process that was both empowering and able to facilitate the change required (Koch and Kralik 2006). It was considered that mixed methods would facilitate a comprehensive understanding of the phenomenon (palliative care delivery) and the context in which it was occurring (residential aged care) (Mertens 2004). Mixed methods was indicated because neither a purely qualitative nor quantitative research paradigm would generate data that would allow exploration, measurement and testing in the setting to address the study questions.

Historical background of action research

The origins of action research are generally attributed to the social psychologist Kurt Lewin, who during the 1940s was concerned with intergroup relations and minority problems (Waterman et al. 2001). Since then researchers from a range of disciplines, including social science, education, psychology and nursing, have contributed to its development (Hart and Bond 1995).

Action research has drawn heavily on critical social science and critical social theory (Reason and Bradbury 2001). As a postpositivist research method, action research is concerned with empowerment (Street 2004). This is in contrast to the positivist framework which seeks to control and contain a phenomenon. Emancipating people from the constraints of irrational, unjust and unproductive forms of life imposed by structures of social dominance and hierarchical structures is the goal of this philosophical framework (Robinson 1999). Action research seeks to empower individuals and organisations to challenge traditional boundaries in respect of methods and, significantly, power relationships (Street 2004). It is concerned with issues surrounding the conduct of empirical research in an unjust world and is driven by an imperative to empower those involved and contribute to the generation of change-enhancing social theory (Winter and Munn-Giddings 2001).

The participatory and democratic process of action research actively involves those who will be affected by the changes. Rather than merely viewing people as the objects of research, action research seeks to engage participants as co-researchers who actively contribute to decision making, enquiry, action and ownership of the outcomes (Badger 2000). The whole purpose of action research is to simultaneously gain an understanding of the social system in order to address the problem, identify the best opportunity for change whilst generating new knowledge about the system (Reason and Bradbury 2001).

Collaborative action is a critical element of this process and helps to bring about change in a situation (Meyer 2000). This requires the researcher to work democratically with and for participants, rather than undertaking research on them. Employing these democratic processes helps to ensure that the research process and outcomes are more meaningful to participants and encourages them to examine and reflect on usual practice (Meyer 2000). Integrating this approach within a mixed methods approach facilitates collaborative problem identification, planning, action and evaluation. This is achieved through using qualitative and quantitative research methods in both exploratory and evaluative contexts and allowing a range of theoretical perspectives that are reconcilable with involvement, empowerment and future orientation.

Relevance of action research to health care

As a consequence of the focus on future orientation and collaboratively working towards a negotiated goal, the approach of action research has been found to be useful in facilitating respectful cooperative and inclusive relationships with health care providers. This is achieved specifically through enabling the naming of problems and identifying of contextually appropriate and sustainable solutions (Williamson and Prosser 2002). In an era of evidence-based practice and clinical governance, engaging health care providers in practice-driven research is increasingly important as it helps to strengthen the nexus between research and usual practice (Cooper and Hewison 2002). Action research can be readily adopted by health care providers concerned with improving the quality of health service delivery (Meyer 2000). Part of the appeal of action research lies in its ability to bridge the gap between theory, research, practice and scientific methods (Elliott 1991). Importantly, action research can positively influence practice while generating data that can be shared with a wider audience and produce tangible benefits (Moyer et al. 1999). Yet, the epistemological basis of action research differs significantly from the traditional sciences in that it aims to produce context-specific and situational knowledge (Winter and Munn-Giddings 2001). Similarly mixed methods research challenges the traditional boundaries of research and is evolving as a novel scientific approach, with its own rigour.

The flexibility of action research has facilitated its use in a variety of natural health and education settings to effect change (Hart and Bond 1995). The cyclical process of action research makes it most appropriate to the needs of organisations wishing to drive change in their environment (Moyer et al. 1999). It is also effective in fostering better practices across inter-professional boundaries and across the care continuum (Meyer 2000). The use of mixed methods within an action research study allows for adaptation of data collection methods to particular settings which assists in better understanding and addressing complex problems (Waterman et al. 2001). This research design is particularly relevant to contemporary health care, where a broad understanding of the complex problems faced in this setting is required to facilitate the development of appropriate practices, services and organisational structures.

Action research's cyclical processes of defining the problem, initiating and evaluating change requires sustained collaboration between researcher and participants, thereby promoting close working relationships and a deeper understanding of the issues involved (Wadsworth 2004). To be effective these action research cycles need to be responsive to events as they naturally occur in the field, which helps ensure that the action is based on democratic processes (Meyer 2000). This approach facilitates the active engagement of participants in the change process and increases the potential for sustainability (Meyer 2000). Success in action research is not evaluated solely on the size of changes made and implementation of solutions, but also from the shared learning that occurs as part of the action research cycle. Therefore the collection of both qualitative and quantitative data can be vital in providing broad outcomes measures. Often novel and unexpected solutions to specific problems emerge from the action research process and these are also important markers of success (Hart and Bond 1995).

Design of the R-PAC Project

The R-PAC Project's eight action research phases utilised mixed methods configured in a sequential transformative design (Mertens 2004). Figure 11.1 illustrates how the action research sequence of reflection, assessment, planning, action and observation supported the transition between the various phases of the R-PAC Project.

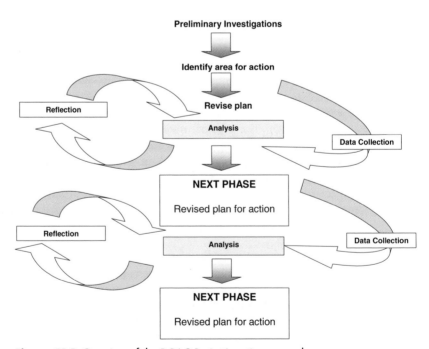

Figure 11.1 Overview of the R-PAC Project's action research process.

Preliminary investigations

Identifying and investigating the problem and exploring the literature was a critical step in this phase of the action research process (Australian Government Department of Health and Ageing 2004). A range of potential change and improvement strategies related to enhancing the delivery of palliative care to older people in the study setting emerged from this process for further consideration.

A needs assessment (Study A) was undertaken as part of the preliminary investigations and included: a critical literature review; review of the epidemiological data; review of relevant policy documents; key informant interviews; and engagement of key stakeholders. This data assisted in identifying the facilitators and barriers to the delivery of best practice palliative care for older people in a rapidly growing regional coastal community in New South Wales (Phillips et al. 2006b). The emergence of paradoxes and contradictions in the preliminary needs assessment data resulted in a reframing of the research questions (Classen and Lopez 2006). Subsequently, the needs assessment became more focused on exploring the palliative care needs of older people in residential aged care. A significant amount of data was collected as part of the focused needs assessment. All data were analysed concurrently with the assistance of the PRECEDE Framework (Green and Kreuter 1991), which allowed for convergence and corroboration of the qualitative and quantitative needs assessment data. During this process, the researcher sought elaboration and clarification of the epidemiological data with findings from the key informant interviews.

During this phase the endorsement and support of key sponsors and stakeholders facilitated the establishment of the Critical Reference Group to guide the development and implementation of the R-PAC Project. The input of a wide cross-section of key stakeholders enhanced the relevance of the enquiry, the meaningfulness of the data and added to the creativity, relevance and effectiveness of the subsequent actions (Wadsworth 2004). Sharing the needs assessment findings with the Critical Reference Group informed the subsequent action research phase and data collection methods. In mixed methods research, this process is known as 'development' and occurs when the results from one method are used to inform the use of another method (Creswell and Plano Clark 2006).

Methodological considerations

Action research was selected as the framework for the R-PAC Project because of the leverage to partner with key stakeholders in the research environment and to engage in collaborative problem solving (Morrison and Lilford 2001). Of significance, this approach offered the potential to ensure that the research processes facilitated opportunities for participants to embrace the social processes of managing and implementing change (Wadsworth 2004). The adoption of action research also ensured that due attention was paid to the subjective meanings for participants and the factors that facilitated a sense of joint ownership of the project's process and outcomes, all of which were identified as being critical for sustainability (Andrew and Halcomb 2006).

The R-PAC Project's action research processes hinged on reflecting on the current situation in order to gain an experiential understanding of the problematic situation and assisted with the generation of the research questions (Johnson and Onwuegbuzie 2004). The specific research questions which the researcher and the critical reference group sought to answer during the R-PAC Project are detailed in Table 11.1. The expansive scope of these research questions suggested that neither purely qualitative nor quantitative methods of data collection would be adequate to provide comprehensive insight into this complex care issue (Mertens 2004). Using mixed methods allowed the researcher to draw from the strengths and minimise the weaknesses of the quantitative and qualitative paradigms across the R-PAC Project's eight sub-studies (Johnson and Onwuegbuzie 2004).

It was also anticipated that conducting a mixed methods research design within an action research framework would help to hasten the teams' understanding of the area of enquiry and achieve the R-PAC Project's research goals in a timely manner (Winter and Munn-Giddings 2001). This occurred because mixed methods offered a practical and outcome-orientated method of enquiry and complemented the action research cycle of reflection, assessment, planning, action and observation. Sharing the data with the Critical Reference Group provided opportunities for a creative period of transformation which enabled new and improved action to be tested (Holter and Schwartz-Barcott 1993). These cyclic processes were repeated until practical considerations, such as time or resources, or achievement of the goals terminated the R-PAC Project.

The decision to use mixed methods in the R-PAC Project triggered a cascade of other methodological considerations. Each of these is discussed in turn below.

Implementation sequence

The R-PAC Project utilised a range of methodological process and data collection methods, some of which were identified prospectively while

Table 11.1 R-PAC research questions and data collection methods.

Research questions	Research method	Study	Phase
(1) What is the current level of palliative care provided to older people in residential aged care in Coffs Harbour, New South Wales?	Focused needs assessment Time 1: Chart audit – End-of-life care	Study A Study B	Preliminary investigations Phase 1
(2) What are the key factors in facilitating palliative care delivery in residential aged care in Coffs Harbour, New South Wales?	Time 1: Focus groups: aged care managers, nurses, care assistants	Study C	Phase 1
(3) What are the major barriers to palliative care delivery to older people in residential aged care in Coffs Harbour, New South Wales?	Time 1: Focus groups: aged care managers, nurses, care assistants	Study C	Phase 1
(4) What are the current palliative care competencies of clinicians working in residential aged care in Coffs Harbour, New South Wales?	Time 1: Survey aged care nurses and care assistants Time 1: Focus groups GPs	Study D Study E	Phase 1 Phase 3
(5) What are the information needs, resources and systems required for the successful delivery of a palliative approach to end-of-life care for residential aged care facilities in a regional community?	Time 2: Focus groups: aged care managers, nurses, care assistants Time 2: Survey aged care nurses and care assistants Time 2: Chart audit – end-of-life care	Study F Study G Study H	Phase 3 Phase 4 Phase 4
(6) What are the key components of a sustainable model of care, to facilitate the delivery of a palliative approach to the end-of-life care for older people in residential aged care in Coffs Harbour, New South Wales?	Model of care development		Phase 5

others were developed with the participants as the action research process unfolded (Creswell and Plano Clark 2006). This resulted in data collection occurring both sequentially (between phases) and concurrently (within phases) within a transformative process (Figure 11.2). The R-PAC Project's sequential data collection occurred between

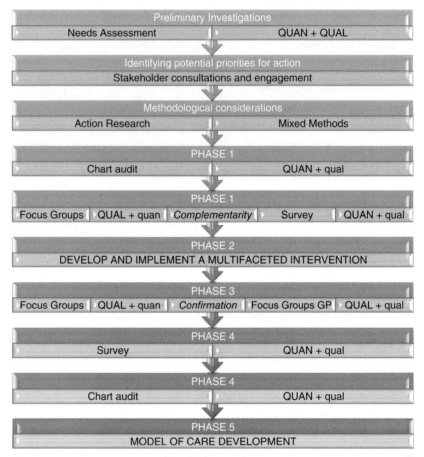

Figure 11.2 Integrating mixed methods into the R-PAC Project's action research framework.

phases, with the data from the previous phase being used to propel the action research process and inform subsequent data collection. Concurrent data collection occurred predominately within the phases, which facilitated a large amount of data to be collected in a relatively short period of time (Morgan 1998).

Priority

In the R-PAC Project, equal emphasis was afforded to both qualitative and quantitative methods to ensure that the R-PAC Project generated data that were in some stages exploratory, while in others focused on process and summative evaluation to drive the process forward

(Johnson and Onwuegbuzie 2004). In adopting this approach the research team realised that the knowledge gained from each dataset had the potential of being either complementary, incommensurate or contradictory (Classen and Lopez 2006). In the context of action research, the emerging of contradictory results is indicative of the need for further exploration and consultation. Thus, the cyclical nature of the action research process helped ensure that what was learnt from each dataset, regardless of whether it was complementary or contradictory, always guided the subsequent phase of the project. Further the use of a mixed methods approach was advantageous in reconciling and validating a range of datasets in sequential and concurrent phases. This engagement ensured that as new knowledge emerged it was acknowledged and addressed. This information then facilitated the research design to evolve in response to the conditions encountered and the information gathered during each phase (Johnson and Onwuegbuzie 2004).

Integration

Mixed methods research is more than just collecting qualitative and quantitative data in the same way that action research is more than an ad hoc collection of disparate processes. Rather mixed methods demands that the data be mixed or integrated, compared, contrasted, appraised and synthesised at some point (Creswell and Plano Clark 2006). The ability to extract adequate information from the data is one of the major rationales for mixed methods data analysis. As previously described, the majority of the R-PAC Project's data was collected and analysed separately in a concurrent (within phase) and sequential design (between phases), with all data from each phase being used to inform the subsequent phase of the action research process (Figure 11.2). The opportunity to integrate different types of data as part of the action research iterative processes was critical to maximising the R-PAC Project's potential whilst also determining its effectiveness.

Theoretical perspective

The R-PAC Project's mixed methods research design was grounded within a transformative paradigm. This paradigm deliberately seeks under-represented populations, gives primacy to value-based and action-orientated dimensions and uses mixed methods to promote change from the personal to the political level (Mertens 2004). In this paradigm, one type of data provides a basis for the collection of another type of data. As the focus is on traditionally underserved groups, sharing the data with participants is an important strategy that enables the group to determine the lessons learnt and identify options for action (Mertens 2004). All of these principles are congruent with those of action research's which involves: active engagement of participants; the establishment of a critical reference group to guide the research process; and utilising the data to drive the action research process through the various cycles of reflecting, planning, acting and evaluating (Street 2004).

Phase One: identifying priorities for action

The key driver during Phase One of the R-PAC Project was to gain greater insight into palliative care delivery in the aged care setting and to further scope the field of enquiry. A prospectively designed chart audit, using selected outcome criteria determined by best practice guidelines, was used to examine the level and type of care provided to residents during the last 72 hours of life prior to the commencement of the R-PAC Project (Time 1) (Study B). The retrospective chart audits were completed by two experienced clinicians. Descriptive statistics were used to analyse the data, with the results confirming that older people dying in residential aged care had unmet palliative care needs. The data revealed that there was scope to enhance the delivery of evidence-based pain management to dying residents and to improve communication with dying residents, their families and other health care providers.

These results were subsequently shared with the Critical Reference Group who recommended that the perceptions of various aged care nurses and care assistants towards palliative care be sought and that a comprehensive assessment of their palliative care competencies be undertaken. A series of focus groups were conducted with aged care management, nurses and care assistants to better understand their perceptions of palliative care delivery and to assist with the identification of facilitators and barriers to palliative care delivery (Study C). Focus group data collection is a form of group interview that generates data through the opinions expressed by participants both individually and collectively (Krueger and Casey 2000). Focus groups were chosen because it is a useful way of developing an understanding of participants' perceptions and feelings about a particular issue, product, service or idea (Phillips et al. 2006a).

The focus groups were conducted by two researchers, with one acting as the facilitator and the other acting as the co-facilitator and scribe. The audio-taped focus group data and field notes were analysed using the process of thematic content analysis (Burnard 1991). The analysis of the transcribed focus group data revealed four broad analytical themes: 1) being like family; 2) advocacy as a key role; 3) communication challenges; and 4) battling and striving to succeed against the odds (Phillips et al. 2006a). These findings demonstrated that aged care nurses and care assistants were committed to providing palliative care to residents but identified the need for greater palliative care competencies and expressed difficulties communicating with other health care providers (Phillips et al. 2006a). Despite the focus group data confirming that aged care staff desired enhanced palliative care competencies, these data didn't identify the domains in which these nurses and care assistants required additional knowledge and skills. Data related to these issues emerged from the survey data.

A survey developed to measure palliative care providers' views and attitudes (Eagar et al. 2003) was selected and administered to a sample of aged care nurses and care assistants in a variety of aged care practice settings (Study D). The quantitative survey data were entered into the Statistical Package for Social Science (SPSS) Version 14.0 to derive descriptive statistics. Chi-squared tests were used to compare the observed and expected frequencies in each category, with $P < 0.05$ being taken to indicate statistical significance (Pallant 2005). The results from the survey corroborated the focus group data that aged care nurses and care assistants expressed the need for greater palliative care competencies but expanded upon this dataset by identifying the specific learning needs each level of health care provider required to develop their palliative care competencies and confidence (Phillips et al. 2007).

The integration of the qualitative and quantitative data at this point facilitated a comprehensive investigation of the level of palliative care provided to older people in residential aged care and enabled the researcher to better understand these phenomena of the facilitators and barriers to palliative care delivery in the aged care setting. These data allowed for the expansion of depth of the enquiry and helped identify the different palliative care learning needs of nurses and care assistants (Phillips et al. 2007). The combination of survey and focus group data collection methods allowed for a process of elaboration and clarification of the results from one dataset with another, which is referred to as 'complementarity' (Creswell and Plano Clark 2006).

Phase Two: developing and implementing the intervention

The use of both qualitative and quantitative data collection methods during Phase One ensured that the researchers obtained a greater understanding of the perceptions of the aged care personnel towards: the delivery of palliative care and their palliative care competencies and level of confidence (Phillips et al., 2008); and the context in which this care was provided (Phillips et al., 2007). This integrated data was fed back to the Critical Reference Group and guided the development of a multifaceted intervention which aimed to enhance the palliative competencies and confidence of aged care nurses and care assistants. The multifaceted intervention was implemented over an 18-month period during Phase Two and involved: implementation of a link nurse role; tailored learning and development strategies; and greater engagement with the specialist palliative care team (Table 11.2).

Phase Three: assessing the impact and seeking direction

At this juncture the Critical Reference Group was keen to assess the impact of the intervention and to seek direction for subsequent action research phases. This need guided the decision to undertake another series of focus groups with aged care providers (Study E) and general practitioners (Study F) to determine their perceptions and impact of the multifaceted intervention. These focus groups were conducted and analysed as two separate studies to allow the values and beliefs of these key groups to be freely disclosed (Wagner et al. 2001).

The data analysis from the aged care provider focus groups revealed four broad analytical themes: 1) targeted education makes a difference; 2) a team approach is valued; 3) assessment tools are helpful; and 4) using the right language is essential (Phillips et al. 2006a). Aged care providers perceived that the multifaceted intervention had enhanced the level of palliative care provided to residents primarily because they felt more confident to: provide palliative care; manage residents' symptoms; and to contact the specialist palliative care team for assistance. Interestingly, greater engagement and understanding of palliative care principles had prompted these aged care staff to desire a more multidisciplinary approach to care planning and delivery (Phillips et al. 2008).

A series of focus groups was undertaken concurrently with general practitioners (GPs) to determine their perceptions of providing a palliative approach to older people in care (Study F). Four key themes emerged from this data: 1) uncertainty about a palliative approach; 2) need to reorientate providers; 3) the challenges of managing third parties; and 4) making it work and moving forward. The focus group data revealed GPs' commitment to caring for older people, wide variability in their understanding of a palliative approach and the

Table 11.2 Summary of R-PAC intervention.

Key elements	Target group	Learning and development strategy	Target
Tailored learning and development intervention	Link nurses	24 hours of palliative skill development workshop 16 hours field placement with the specialist palliative care team 2 hour bi-monthly peer support meetings Option to enrol in an accredited palliative care module and receive 10 credit points towards a postgraduate diploma in palliative care nursing	1 link nurse per 50 aged care beds
	Registered nurses	2 day palliative care skill development workshop	1 additional registered nurse per aged care facility
	Care assistants	16 hours palliative care skill development workshop Opportunity to network with other care assistants from local residential aged care facility Opportunity to meet with: Specialist Palliative Care Team and Aged Care Assessment Team, and link nurse from their aged care facility	150 care assistants
	General practitioners	8 hour palliative care field placement with the specialist palliative care team, including attending the multidisciplinary care planning meeting, specialist outpatient clinic and home visits	22 general practitioners
Participation in specialist palliative care multi-agency, multidisciplinary team meeting	Link nurses, registered nurses, general practitioners	Attendance at the multidisciplinary team meeting during all field placements Action learning opportunities Networking opportunities Opportunity for residents with complex palliative care needs to have their care planned by the multidisciplinary team	All link nurses and general practitioners

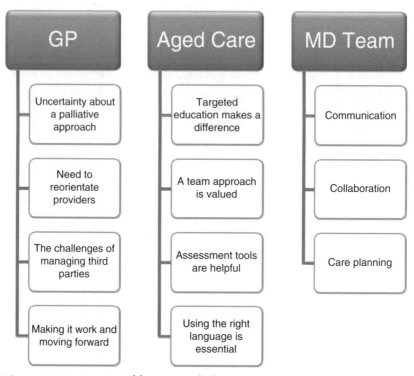

Figure 11.3 Integration of focus group findings.

challenges of integrating the demands of aged care into their busy work schedules. A number of options, including the establishing of multi-disciplinary care planning, were proposed to facilitate a more systematic approach to care delivery for older people.

Following the analysis of these datasets, individual data were compared to elucidate common issues and concerns, which are summarised in Figure 11.3. The common issues which emerged relate to the creation of multidisciplinary teams as a vehicle to enhance communication, collaboration and care planning.

Sharing these findings with participants and the Critical Reference Group helped set the direction for the subsequent phase of the action research process: trialling of in-house weekly multidisciplinary team meetings in four residential aged care facilities and the collaborative development of a palliative approach information pamphlet.

Phase Four: measuring the impact

In order to further validate the perception of aged care nurses and care assistants that they had greater palliative care competencies and felt more confident in negotiating residents' care a decision was made by the Critical Reference Group to repeat the survey and chart audits instruments used in Phase One. This decision allowed for the effect of the multifaceted intervention to be measured using a non-equivalent group pre-test–post-test research design. This is a common tool used in social research to compare the impact of an intervention and is structured in a pre-test–post-test manner using intact groups (Polit and Beck 2006). The absence of a control group limits the ability confidently to attribute changes to an intervention. In spite of these limitations, this process is common to action research projects as the philosophical underpinnings are not driven by a positivist framework of testing (Reason and Bradbury 2001). Rather, action research adopts processes to foster a collaborative approach to negotiate goals using a range of enabling strategies. For this reason a non-equivalent group design is used extensively in quality improvement projects (Ovretveit and Gustafson 2002) and collaborative methodology (Wilson et al. 2003) as it can both measure the impact of interventions and drive ongoing clinical improvement.

Within the R-PAC Project (Table 11.1), the pre-test and post-test study groups consisted of two discrete study populations: registered nurses and care assistants employed in residential aged care responsible for the delivery of patient care in 2004 (Pre-test, Time 1) and in 2006 (Post-test, Time 2) (Study G); and residents who had died in 2003 (Pre-test, Time 1) and in 2005 (Post-test, Time 2) (Study H).

The findings from the Time 2 survey data revealed greater levels of palliative care confidence and competencies for all levels of aged care providers, with higher confidence levels found amongst care assistants. The descriptive statistics showed an increasing trend at Time 2 towards a more appropriate use of palliative care medications, enhanced communication with families and greater specialist palliative care input to residents with complex care needs. Despite this trend towards improved palliative care delivery for dying residents at Time 2, the data also revealed limited utilisation of pain assessment tools and low levels of advance care planning.

These results were shared with the Critical Reference Group who felt that the contradictions in the chart audit data posed a series of new research questions (Koch and Kralik 2001), to be explored in subsequent action research cycles.

Phase Five: developing the model of care

The data collected throughout the R-PAC Project informed the collaborative development of a model of care to promote the delivery of a palliative approach in residential aged care. It was at this stage that the cumulative findings and data afforded through the mixed methods approach were all synthesised and interpreted.

The use of action research and mixed methods demonstrated the effectiveness of engaging aged care providers in a change process aimed at embedding a palliative approach in residential aged care. The data provided valuable insights into how to improve the delivery of palliative care with the findings from the substudies being used to propel the action research process and forming the basis of the proposed model of care. This model acknowledges that death is an expected occurrence for older people living in residential aged care and challenges policy makers and health care planners to ensure that a palliative approach underpins all future aged care policy development and is funded accordingly. Integral to this model is a commitment to ongoing learning and development interventions, and adoption of a multidisciplinary approach to care planning and delivery to ensure that the needs of residents and their families are adequately addressed.

Challenges for the novice researcher

Mastering mixed methods research is not without its challenges and limitations. Utilising mixed methods within action research adds to the complexity of the research process. This is amplified by the inherent challenges associated with conducting and reporting action research's dynamic processes (Whyte et al. 1991). Being an exploratory process, action research needs to be responsive to contexts, rather than being prescriptive in its measures and processes and this requires preparedness from the researcher that their relationship with participants will be dynamic and likely to undergo continuous evolution. Significantly, it relies on the researcher tolerating ambiguity and uncertainty and accepting that the action research journey and its final destination are somewhat unknown. During this journey the researcher is often challenged by events, ideas, information and arguments and reconciling various paradigms (Johnson and Turner 2003). Managing this requires a flexible stance and an ability to cope with conducting research in dynamic clinical areas where things are constantly undergoing rapid change.

A significant amount of data was collected during each phase of the R-PAC Project's action research process which required a management system to deal with qualitative, quantitative and integrated data. The utilisation of mixed methods also required the researchers to have a sound understanding of the defining characteristics, strengths and weaknesses of both quantitative and qualitative paradigms. Developing these competencies takes considerable time, effort and experience, all of which makes a collaborative research approach a prerequisite for utilising mixed methods. Unfortunately, this resource requirement is a major barrier to employing mixed methods. Prior to embarking on a mixed methods study the research team needs to have addressed these limitations to maximise the potential of the researcher to mix or combine data collection strategies, which is the fundamental principle of mixed methods research. In addition, it is often challenging to disseminate the complexity of mixed method approaches within the word limits of many peer-reviewed journals.

Conclusion

The R-PAC Project's use of mixed methods within action research allowed for the exploration of palliative care delivery, from a multifaceted perspective, in residential aged care and the formulation of strategies to improve future care. Study sequences were adopted according to the research questions and direction of the action research process, the theoretical and methodological considerations and the need to integrate these perspectives and allow interpretation within the research team. In the conduct and design of the project, qualitative and quantitative data were considered to be of equal significance and importance and followed an action research sequence. In spite of the philosophical differences of the quantitative and qualitative paradigms, the use of mixed methods generated a rich and lucrative data source, informing the direction and facilitating process and summative evaluation. The use of action research allowed for a dynamic, iterative, inclusive and reflective framework to improve the care of residents as well as addressing a range of nurses' and care assistants' personal and professional issues, demonstrating that mechanisms that promote ownership and control over circumstances are more likely to drive health care reform and promote sustainability in contemporary health care settings.

Key points

- Action research is a future-orientated process focusing on collaboration, empowerment and reform which makes it well suited to the complex environment of contemporary health care systems.
- Mixed methods is well accommodated within the dynamic contents of action research.

- Adherence to methodological rigour is important from the perspective of both mixed methods and action research.
- Incorporating a range of methodological perspectives requires a suite of skills in qualitative and quantitative methods.

References

Andrew S. and Halcomb E.J. (2006) Mixed methods research is an effective method of enquiry for community health research. *Contemporary Nurse*, **23**, 145–153.

Australian Department of Health and Ageing and National Health and Medical Research Council (2006) *Guidelines for a Palliative Approach in Residential Aged Care – enhanced version*. Canberra, ACT.

Australian Government Department of Health and Ageing (2004) *Guidelines for a Palliative Approach in Residential Aged Care*. Canberra, ACT.

Australian Institute of Health and Welfare (2004) *Residential Aged Care in Australia 2002–03: A Statistical Overview*. Canberra, ACT: Australian Institute of Health and Welfare.

Badger T.G. (2000) Action research, change and methodological rigour. *Journal of Nursing Management*, **8**, 201–207.

Burnard P. (1991) A method of analysing interview transcripts in qualitative research. *Nurse Education Today*, **11**, 461–466.

Classen S. and Lopez E.D.S. (2006) Mixed methods approach explaining process of an older driver safety systematic review. *Topics in Geriatric Rehabilitation*, **22**, 99–122.

Commonwealth Department of Health and Aged Care (1997) *Aged Care Act*. Canberra, ACT.

Cooper J. and Hewison A. (2002) Implementing audit in palliative care: an action research approach. *Journal of Advanced Nursing*, **39**, 360–369.

Creswell J.W. and Plano Clark V. (2006) *Designing and Conducting Mixed Methods Research*. Thousand Oaks, California: Sage Publications.

Currow D.C. and Hegarty M. (2006) Residential aged care facility palliative care guidelines: Improving care. *International Journal of Palliative Nursing*, **12**, 231–233.

Davies E. and Higginson I. (2004) *Better Palliative Care for Older People*. Copenhagen: World Health Organization.

Eagar K., Senior K., Fildes D., Quinsey K., Owen A., Yeatman H. et al. (2003) *The Rural Palliative Care Evaluation Tool Kit: A Compendium of Tools to Aid in the Evaluation of Palliative Care Projects*. Wollongong, NSW. University of Wollongong Centre Health Services Development.

Elliott J. (1991) *Action Research for Educational Change*. Buckingham: Open University Press.

Green L.W. and Kreuter M.W. (1991) *Health Promotion Planning: An Educational and Environmental Approach*. Mountain View, California: Mayfield Publishing Company.

Hart E. and Bond M. (1995) *Action Research for Health and Social Care: A Guide to Practice.* Buckingham: Open University Press.

Holter M.I. and Schwartz-Barcott D. (1993) Action research: what is it? How has it been used and how can it be used in nursing? *Journal of Advanced Nursing*, **18**, 298–304.

Johnson B. and Turner L.A. (2003) Data collection strategies in mixed methods research. In Tashakkori A. and Teddlie C. (eds.) *Handbook of Mixed Methods in Social and Behavioral Research*, 2nd edition, pp. 297–319. Thousand Oaks, California: Sage Publications.

Johnson R.B. and Onwuegbuzie A.J. (2004) Mixed method research: a research paradigm whose time has come. *Educational Researcher*, **33**, 14–26.

Koch T. and Kralik D. (2001) Chronic illness: reflections on a community-based action research programme. *Journal of Advanced Nursing*, **36**, 23–31.

Koch T. and Kralik D. (2006) *Participatory Action Research in Health Care.* Oxford: Blackwell Publishers.

Krueger R.A. and Casey M.A. (2000) *Focus Groups: A Practical Guide for Applied Research.* Thousand Oaks, California: Sage Publications.

Mertens D. (2004) *Research and Evaluation in Education and Psychology: Integrating Diversity with Quantitative, Qualitative, and Mixed Methods.* Thousand Oaks, California: Sage Publications.

Meyer J. (2000) Using qualitative methods in health related action research. *British Medical Journal*, **320**, 178–181.

Morgan D.L. (1998) Practical strategies for combining qualitative and quantitative methods: applications to health research. *Qualitative Health Research*, **8**, 362–376.

Morrison B. and Lilford R.J. (2001) How can action research apply to health services? *Qualitative Health Research*, **11**, 436–449.

Moyer A., Corstine M., Jamault M., Roberge G. and O'Hagan M. (1999) Identifying older people in need using action research. *Journal of Clinical Nursing*, **8**, 103–111.

Ovretveit J. and Gustafson D. (2002) Evaluation of quality improvement programmes. *Quality and Safety in Health Care*, **11**, 270–275.

Pallant J. (2005) *SPSS Survival Manual: a Step by Step Guide to Data Analysis Using SPSS.* Sydney: Allen and Unwin.

Phillips J. (2007) *Navigating a Palliative Approach in Residential Aged Care Using a Population Based Approach.* Sydney: University of Western Sydney.

Phillips J., Davidson P., Kristjanson L., Jackson D. and Daly J. (2006a) Residential aged care: the last frontier for palliative care. *Journal of Advanced Nursing*, **55**, 416–424.

Phillips J.L., Davidson P.M., Jackson D., Kristjanson L., Bennett M.L. and Daly J. (2006b) Enhancing palliative care delivery in a regional community in Australia. *Australian Health Review*, **30**, 370–379.

Phillips J.L., Davidson P.M., Jackson D. and Kristjanson L.J. (2008) Multi-faceted palliative care intervention: aged care nurses' and care assistants' perceptions and experiences. *Journal of Advanced Nursing*, **62**(2), 216–227.

Phillips J.L., Davidson P.M., Ollerton R., Jackson D. and Kristjanson L. (2007) Commitment and compassion: survey results from nurses and care assistants working in residential aged care. *International Journal of Palliative Nursing*, **13**(6), 282–290.

Polit D.F. and Beck C.T. (2006) *Essentials of Nursing Research: Methods, Appraisal and Utilization.* Philadelphia: Lippincott Williams and Wilkins.

Reason P. and Bradbury H. (2001) *Handbook of Action Research.* London: Sage Publications.

Robinson A. (1999) At the interface of health and community care: developing linkages between aged care services in a rural context. *Australian Journal of Rural Health*, **7**, 172–180.

Royal Australian College of General Practitioners (2006) *Medical Care of Older Persons in Residential Aged Care Facilities.* Melbourne, Australia: Royal Australian College of General Practitioners.

Street A. (2004) Action Research. In Minichiello V., Sullivan G., Greenwood K. and Axford R. (eds.) *Research Methods for Nursing and Health Science,* 2nd edition, pp. 278–294. Sydney: Pearson Education Australia.

Wadsworth Y. (2004) *Everyday Evaluation on the Run.* Sydney: Allen and Unwin.

Wagner E.H., Glasgow R.E., Davis C., Bonomi A.E., Provost L., McCulloch D. et al. (2001) Quality improvement in chronic illness care: a collaborative approach. *Joint Commission Journal on Quality Improvement*, **27**, 63–80.

Wasson K. (2000) Ethical arguments for providing palliative care to non-cancer patients. *International Journal of Palliative Nursing*, **6**, 66–70.

Waterman H.A., Tillen D., Dickson R. and de Koning K. (2001) Action research: a systematic review and guidance for assessment. *Health Technology Assessment*, **5**, iii–157. http://www.hta.ac.uk/fullmono/mon523.pdf

Whyte W.F., Greenwood D.J. and Lazes P. (eds.) (1991) *Participatory Action Research.* Newbury Park, CA: Sage Publications.

Williamson G.R. and Prosser S. (2002) Action research: politics, ethics and participation. *Journal of Advanced Nursing*, **40**, 587–593.

Wilson T., Berwick D.M. and Cleary P.D. (2003) What do collaborative improvement projects do? Experience from seven countries. *Joint Commission Journal on Quality and Safety*, **29**, 85–93.

Winter R. and Munn-Giddings C. (2001) *Handbook for Action Research in Health and Social Care.* London: Routledge.

Future Challenges for Mixed Methods Research in Nursing and the Health Sciences

Sharon Andrew and Elizabeth J. Halcomb

Introduction

Nursing and health science researchers have, increasingly, embraced mixed methods to guide their exploration of the complex phenomena that influence human health. The mixed methods approach offers a flexibility and depth of insight that is not possible to achieve through the use of either qualitative or quantitative methods alone. Despite a growth in popularity, it is clear to us that using mixed methods approaches in themselves does not mean that the research is inherently good. High quality application of the mixed methods approach requires consideration of the theoretical underpinnings and careful planning of data collection methods and analysis techniques. Like its qualitative and quantitative counterparts, the mixed methods approach can be of variable quality and rigour. In order to maintain the integrity of mixed methods as a research approach it is vital that researchers engage in scholarly debate within the literature not only regarding philosophical issues, but also practical considerations, to guide those using mixed methods in their research. This text has sought to do this by providing a combination of practical advice supplemented with contemporary examples from the literature and introducing the reader to the current issues faced by nursing and the health science researchers using mixed methods.

This chapter will highlight key issues related to the development of mixed methods that have been raised throughout the text. By doing this we hope that this chapter will provide the impetus for more scholarly debate in the evolution of mixed methods research in nursing and the health sciences.

Paradigmatic issues for mixed methods: moving forwards

Twinn (2003) was perhaps overly optimistic when she stated that, on the basis of increased nursing studies in the literature and material included in nursing textbooks, mixed methods is now accepted in nursing and the 'paradigm wars have been resolved' (p. 549). There certainly has been a shift from scepticism (Rossman and Wilson 1985; Leininger 1994) to acceptance in nursing (Flemming 2007) and other health sciences (Whitley 2007). There is less open warfare, and the question 'Is it possible?' has been replaced by others such 'How can we conduct mixed methods research and retain rigour?' and 'Is mixed methods a paradigm?' This change may be in part due to the fact that while theorists were debating whether it was possible to mix data, researchers in the field were forging ahead and conducting studies using mixed methods in a variety of clinical, academic and policy settings. In essence, the practice of health researchers has driven the agenda for the development of mixed methods.

Pragmatism has been advanced as a practical theoretical underpinning for mixed methods. Some of the questions that are hindering the advancement of the paradigm issue are discussed in Chapter 2 by Muncey and in the recent literature (Giddings 2006; Giddings and Grant 2007; Morgan 2007; Greene 2008). The discourse in this area needs to be intensified if theory is to keep pace with research practice. Examining the mixed methods studies that have been published in the peer-reviewed literature, as undertaken by O'Cathain (Chapter 8) or Creswell and colleagues (Chapter 9), may assist in the development of theory that is based on actual mixed methods research. In order to maintain the integrity of mixed methods research, it is vital that philosophical and theoretical underpinnings guide research practice.

We believe that this text will support and advance the recognition of mixed methods research as a separate paradigm. We agree that mixed methods researchers need to assist this recognition by continued scholarly debate, and increased publication of theoretical discourse about the issues that underpin the paradigm debate. Our ideal situation would be to have nursing and health researchers halting any arguments about whether mixed methods is a separate paradigm, accept that it is, albeit in early stages, and advance its development in a united fashion.

Research designs and mixed methods

The continued debate about mixed methods and whether it is a separate paradigm is likely to linger for some time. However, acceptance of a new paradigm that incorporates mixed methods is a key step in moving forward and shaping how mixed methods research is conceptualised and approached. Researchers conducting mixed methods research are challenged to consider how their research design might add to our understanding of the theoretical underpinnings of mixed methods research. For example, publishing their study in its entirety, including outlining how the problem, research question(s), research design and data analysis including integration were conducted, will assist others conducting similar studies. This may limit what is described as 'cherry-picking' (Whitley 2007) key qualitative and quantitative findings for separate specialist journals thus avoiding the description of the study in its entirety. While in recent years specific methodological journals have emerged for mixed methods research (*Journal of Mixed Methods*; *International Journal of Multiple Research Approaches*), these publications remain in their infancy and still do not contain detailed reports of both the methodological aspects and study findings. Consideration should be given to how such publications can advance the development of the mixed methods approach without diluting the dissemination of important findings in speciality clinical practice journals.

One area that has disappointed researchers is the description of how data are integrated. In our experience, whether presenting papers at conferences or in the peer-reviewed literature, researchers tend to avoid the hard questions of how they integrated their data. Discussion of this area is often neglected with researchers skipping to results with no mention of how their data were combined. Bazeley (Chapter 6) is leading the field in developing ways of mixing data, particularly through the use of computer software. Others must join the discourse and describe the processes of integration that they have used in their investigations within research reports. This description may also enhance the assessment of the rigour of a mixed methods study.

Kroll and Neri outline the common mixed methods designs in Chapter 3 and, in Chapter 8, O'Cathain expands on this in her discussion of the many designs identified in health research. The examples discussed in Chapters 9–11 also add to our understanding of how mixed methods research designs may be adapted to suit clinical research problems in nursing and the health sciences.

In Chapter 11, Phillips and Davidson have outlined how an action research study used a mixed methods approach. This description adds to the debate about mixed methods research designs and the way that they may be viewed differently by different researchers. Participatory action research can be viewed from the perspective of mixed methods as incorporating a transformative design (Mertens 2003) whereas others do not link this method to mixed methods *per se* (Koch and Kralik 2006). More discourse is clearly required about how and where this and other designs, such as case study, ethnography and evaluation studies, are situated within mixed methods. For example, should they be 'slotted' into the common designs identified in Chapter 3 or should they be described separately? In this text we have tended to do the latter but recognise the need for continuing discourse about this issue.

Reflexivity and the mixed methods researcher

At present there are few 'true' mixed methodologists; that is, research-ers who have specialist education in mixed methods research including its design, conduct and the integration of data. While some higher education institutions offer courses in mixed methods research, we expect that, like us, many researchers have come from more traditional research education with a specialism in a specific methodological approach. The use of mixed methods among those who have under-gone this education indicates a degree of flexibility and acceptance of working outside the traditional boundaries of a methodology. Never-theless, we must recognise that our education into a predominant para-digm has influenced how we view and conduct research. Moreover, even if we undergo additional training or education in another meth-odology, we may not necessarily be 'experts' in this methodology com-pared to the one in which we were predominantly prepared. We must accept therefore that our view of a mixed methods problem may be framed by our educational background and other aspects that comprise us, namely our personal, social and cultural backgrounds (Morgan 2007). Until there is a mixed methodologist we believe that persons doing mixed methods research should apply what Giddings and Grant (Chapter 7) refer to as self-reflexivity by identifying their educational background that may influence their perception of a research problem so the reader can determine for themselves the pragmatism of their approach.

The mixed methodologist

Historically, researchers have been dichotomised as being primarily qualitative or quantitative in their research programmes. The emergence of mixed methods has created the need for a new genre of researcher, the mixed methodologist. Currently researchers often enter the field of mixed methods with past experience in either the qualitative or quantitative paradigm, but future researchers may commence their research career from a mixed methods perspective. These individuals will not have the same influences from their background as those who have long espoused either the qualitative or quantitative approach and then moved into mixed methods research. Pure mixed methodologists will, like their qualitative and quantitative counterparts, be erudite into a specific paradigm which describes their ontological and epistemological positions and guides their research programme.

The mixed methodologist is not a 'Jack of all trades'. As the field of mixed methods continues to develop, these individuals will be highly skilled researchers in their own right with a unique and highly valuable skill set. These researchers will need to understand positivism, naturalism and pragmatism, as well as their implications for research design, data collection and analysis. As it is probably not possible to have high-level data collection and analysis skills in both qualitative and quantitative approaches, the mixed methodologist must have adequate team management and interpersonal skills to convene and facilitate a team comprising of expert researchers from the various paradigms. In terms of their own unique skills, the mixed methodologist must have expertise in the integration and mixing aspects of the study. Currently, this aspect of conducting mixed methods research is somewhat invisible. Future work needs to explore, expand and test innovative ways of truly combining qualitative and quantitative data to achieve the intended purposes of mixed methods enquiry.

Research training

The mixed methodologists of the future may evolve from current candidates of doctoral and master's programmes. Higher degree research candidature is the perfect opportunity to facilitate high-level skill development in relation to philosophical and methodological approaches to research. Mixed methods designs can lend themselves well to doctoral and master's programmes as they can involve a series of relatively smaller data collections that can provide a deeper insight, and are often easier to manage than a single larger collection. Despite this potential, many candidates conducting what are reported as mixed methods studies do not receive supervision from academics skilled specifically in mixed methods approaches. This is occurring for a number of reasons. Firstly, although it is generally accepted that mixed methods is growing in popularity in nursing and the health sciences, few academics recognise the specialist expertise required to conduct high-quality mixed methods research. Whilst it would be unthinkable to have a doctoral student conducting a quantitative study without at least one supervisor having expertise in quantitative methodology, many doctoral students conducting mixed methods investigations have no members of the supervision panel with mixed methods expertise. In this way, mixed methods is still not considered a specialist methodological approach akin to qualitative or quantitative approaches. Without a supervisor to provide specialist discourse, the student is left to struggle with the philosophical issues, design considerations and the practical aspects of integrating qualitative and quantitative data. For many, as has been highlighted in Chapter 6, this may result in suboptimal application of the approach to address their research problem. Supervision panels consisting of a combination of qualitative and quantitative experts may experience problems related to the diametrically opposing views of the supervisors about how the project should proceed. Without adequate mediation, these supervision panels can impact significantly on the progress of the student and the quality of their work.

Secondly, as mixed methods research remains in its adolescence, there are limited numbers of researchers who have high-level expertise in this approach and can offer supervision to higher degree research candidates. Whilst many researchers may report expertise in mixed methods after having conducted a small number of mixed methods enquiries, one could argue that true expertise involves not only practical experience, but also participation in the scholarly discourse and development of the approach.

Despite these challenges, it is vital to the future development of mixed methods that upcoming researchers are provided with appropriate training to facilitate both their own professional growth and their potential to contribute to the development of mixed methods research.

Evidence-based practice

Mixed methods research clearly has an important role in the developing evidence-based health care movement. Whilst randomised controlled trials have been traditionally considered the gold standard, mixed methods offers a broader approach to best practice that is inclusive of considerations such as consumer perceptions, community values and issues of evidence transfer and implementation. The scope of mixed methods extends beyond simply their utility in intervention trials, as we have seen in Chapter 9, and encompasses a range of research designs that can address the complex health problems that face our society in the environment of ageing and chronic disease. The use of a mixed methods approach increases the potential for the evidence generated to be directly applicable to practitioners within the clinical context (Flemming 2007). Enhancing the applicability of evidence increases the probability of its implementation into practice by clinicians, managers and policy makers (Flemming 2007).

Before mixed methods can truly be accepted as a conventional source of evidence, however, standardised appraisal guidelines and tools need to be developed. As has been demonstrated by Giddings and Grant in Chapter 7, measuring the quality of mixed methods research is more than simply evaluating the various components using traditional measures of validity and rigour. The issue of quality appraisal for mixed methods research needs to be the subject of future scholarly discourse and debate to ensure that a robust mechanism is developed to support the appropriate critical appraisal of this growing body of research.

Conclusion

It is exciting and a unique opportunity to be able to contribute to the development of mixed methods research. Whilst there is increasing acceptance of this approach to enquiry in nursing and the health sciences, future developments in the field need to be undertaken strategically and in a scholarly fashion to ensure that the quality of approach is maintained and innovation in design and analysis approaches is fostered. Greater discourse needs to focus not only on paradigmatic and design issues, but also on the practical issues of implementing mixed methods in clinical research and achieving true integration of qualitative and quantitative datasets. Additionally, the development of mixed methodologists and the training of emerging researchers needs to be further examined.

References

Flemming K. (2007) The knowledge base for evidence-based nursing: A role for mixed methods research? *Advances in Nursing Science*, **30**, 41–51.

Giddings L.S. (2006) Mixed-methods research: positivism dressed in drag? *Journal of Research in Nursing*, **11**, 195–203.

Giddings L.S. and Grant B.M. (2007) A Trojan Horse for positivism? A critique of mixed methods research. *Advances in Nursing Science*, **30**, 52–60.

Greene J.C. (2008) Is mixed methods social inquiry a distinctive methodology? *Journal of Mixed Methods Research*, **2**, 7–22.

Koch T. and Kralik D. (2006) *Participatory Action Research in Health Care*. Oxford: Blackwell Publishing Ltd.

Leininger M.M. (1994) Evaluation criteria and critique of qualitative research studies. In Morse J.M. (ed.) *Critical Issues in Qualitative Research Methods*, pp. 95–115. Thousand Oaks: Sage Publications.

Mertens D.M. (2003) Mixed methods and the politics of human research: the transformative-emancipatory perspective. In Tashakkori A. and Teddlie C. (eds.) *Handbook of Mixed Methods in Social and Behavioral Research*, pp. 135–164. Thousand Oaks: Sage Publications.

Morgan D.L. (2007) Paradigms lost and pragmatism regained: methodological implications of combining qualitative and quantitative methods. *Journal of Mixed Methods Research*, **1**, 48–76.

Rossman G.B. and Wilson B.L. (1985) Numbers and words: combining quantitative and qualitative methods in a single large-scale evaluation study. *Evaluation Review*, **9**, 627–643.

Twinn S. (2003) Status of mixed methods in research in nursing. In Tashakkori A. and Teddlie C. (eds.) *Handbook of Mixed Methods in Social and Behavioral Research*, pp. 541–556. Thousand Oaks: Sage Publications.

Whitley R. (2007) Mixed-methods studies. *Journal of Mental Health*, **16**, 697–701.

Index